STATIC CONTRACTION
TRAINING

About the Authors

Peter Sisco is the coauthor of *Power Factor Training* (Contemporary Books) and the innovator of the Power Factor and Power Index methods of measuring muscular overload. His articles have appeared in every major bodybuilding publication in America and in many foreign countries. He is also the coauthor of *The Golfer's Two-Minute Workout* (Contemporary Books), *Power Factor Specialization: Chest and Arms* (Contemporary Books, Spring 1999), and the editor of *Ironman's Ultimate Bodybuilding Encyclopedia* (Contemporary Books, Summer 1999).

John R. Little's articles have been published in every martial arts and health and fitness magazine in America. He is the author of *The Warrior Within* and *Bruce Lee: Words from a Master* (Contemporary Books), the coauthor of *Power Factor Training*, *The Golfer's Two-Minute Workout* (Contemporary Books), and *Power Factor Specialization: Chest and Arms* (Contemporary Books, Spring 1999), and the innovator of the static contraction method of strength training. In addition, Little is the editor of the twelve-volume *Bruce Lee Library Series* (Charles E. Tuttle Publishing) and the five-volume *Inside Kung Fu Library Series*. Little spent his formative years in Agincourt and Muskoka and received his B.A. from McMaster University in Hamilton, Ontario. He is happily married and the proud father of three children.

STATIC CONTRACTION TRAINING

Gain Up to 25 Pounds of Pure Muscle Mass in 10 Weeks!

Peter Sisco and John R. Little

CB
CONTEMPORARY BOOKS

Library of Congress Cataloging-in-Publication Data

Sisco, Peter.
      Static contraction training : gain up to 25 pounds of pure
muscle mass in 10 weeks / Peter Sisco and John Little.
            p.   cm.
      ISBN 0-8092-2907-2
      1. Bodybuilding—Physiological aspects.   2. Muscle tone.
3. Muscle strength.   4. Muscle contraction.   I. Little, John R.,
1960–   .   II. Title.
RC1235.S57   1998
646.7′5—dc21   98–7262
                                                                   CIP

Cover design by Todd Petersen
Cover and interior photographs copyright © Mitsuru Okabe Company.
Interior design by Hespenheide Design

Published by Contemporary Books
A division of NTC/Contemporary Publishing Group, Inc.
4255 West Touhy Avenue, Lincolnwood (Chicago), Illinois 60646-1975 U.S.A.
Copyright © 1999 by Peter Sisco and John R. Little
Printed in the United States of America
International Standard Book Number: 0-8092-2907-2
  99   00   01   02   03   VL   6   5   4   3   2   1

This book is dedicated to every person who is willing to apply reason, logic, and the scientific method to discover truth. From Empedocles to Galileo to, perhaps, the person holding this book, these are the people who insist on evidence, eschew dogma, help discover new knowledge, and thereby improve the lives of all.

PETER SISCO

To a very boring logic professor from northern Ontario whose bromidic lectures caused me to daydream. For it was during one such reverie that Static Contraction Training was born, thus proving the value—however serendipitous—of a formal education.

JOHN R. LITTLE

Caution: This program involves a systematic progression of muscular overload that leads to the lifting of extremely heavy weights. As a result, a proper warm-up of muscles, tendons, ligaments, and joints is mandatory at the beginning of every workout.

Warning: As this is a very intense program, it requires both a thorough knowledge of proper exercise form and a base level of strength fitness. Although exercise is very beneficial, the potential for injury does exist, especially if the trainee is not in good physical condition. Always consult with your physician before beginning any program of progressive weight training or exercise. If you feel any strain or pain when you are exercising, stop immediately and consult your physician.

Contents

Foreword

More than 30 years ago, as a teenager in search of more muscle, I decided to make a greater commitment to my training and give it everything I had. I abandoned the program I was doing two to three times per week that revolved around squats, pullovers, overhead presses, chins, and dips and embarked on a much more ambitious program. Following the conventional wisdom of the time and emulating some well-known physique stars, I began a program involving 15 to 20 sets per body part and six training sessions per week. Overall, I was doing about 300 sets per week and training almost 15 hours.

This foray into "advanced" training didn't last very long. I recall being constantly sick and dreading most of the monotonous workouts. I eventually returned to my more "modest" workouts and made some outstanding gains.

At that time I just wasn't smart enough to grasp, let alone fully understand, what my experience should have told me about the principles of effective training. My mind was still fixated on the notion that the more sets I could do and the more pumped up I could get—if somehow I could stay pumped up all the time—the bigger and stronger I would get. Graduate school, a professional career, and other interests always precluded returning to that ultimate "advanced" routine. Time constraints and some real sense that I just couldn't do very high-volume training generally kept me following what today would be considered a fairly basic high-intensity training program consisting of 15 to 20 sets performed three to four times per week. This training was always accompanied by running several days per week and then later by various other types of cardiovascular training. I modestly improved on this type of schedule, but I was constantly tired and sore.

Scientific principles, the writings of others, and my own experience suggested that there must be logical next steps that could make my training even more efficient and effective. For example, it's likely that focusing my training on a handful of basic movements and reducing the frequency of my cardiovascular training could increase my strength and cardiovascular fitness—quite a turnaround from my weeks of performing 300 sets!

Static Contraction Training, pioneered by Pete Sisco and John Little, is an emerging, innovative system of training that capitalizes on the principles of high-intensity training and applies them in a logical, exciting way. This book shows how it is possible to dramatically increase strength and muscle mass using static contractions in a very limited number of movements. Training that was once thought to require many hours per week might now be done in minutes per week.

Sisco and Little, much to their credit, would be the first to say that more needs to be learned about Static Contraction Training. What exactly is the best protocol? What is the precise relationship between gains in static contraction strength and dynamic strength? You must also follow the rules and guidelines for Static Contraction Training regarding charting progress, regulating overload, and the volume and frequency of training. Adherence to all safety measures is important because Static Contraction Training typically involves using a great deal of resistance in your strongest position. As with any system of training, you can only progress if you remain injury free.

Sisco and Little do not promise that Static Contraction Training will make you an overnight physique sensation or an instant world-class strength athlete. What they do promise is a great opportunity to try a totally innovative training system and be part of a grand experiment that is moving bodybuilding and strength training toward a new paradigm of efficiency.

RICHARD A. WINETT, PH.D.

Acknowledgments

We wish to thank master physique photographer Mitsuru Okabe for all of the photographs in this book.

Special thanks to Gold's Gym in Boise, Idaho, for generously allowing us to use its facilities during the photographing of exercises and to Mike Reed and Todd Opheim for posing for some of the photos.

We also wish to thank Richard Winett, Ph.D., for his kind words in the foreword to this book and for being among the very first to promote Static Contraction Training in his excellent newsletter, *Master Trainer* (www.agelessathletes.com). Dr. Winett has been among the few voices of rationality and science in the field of bodybuilding and strength training.

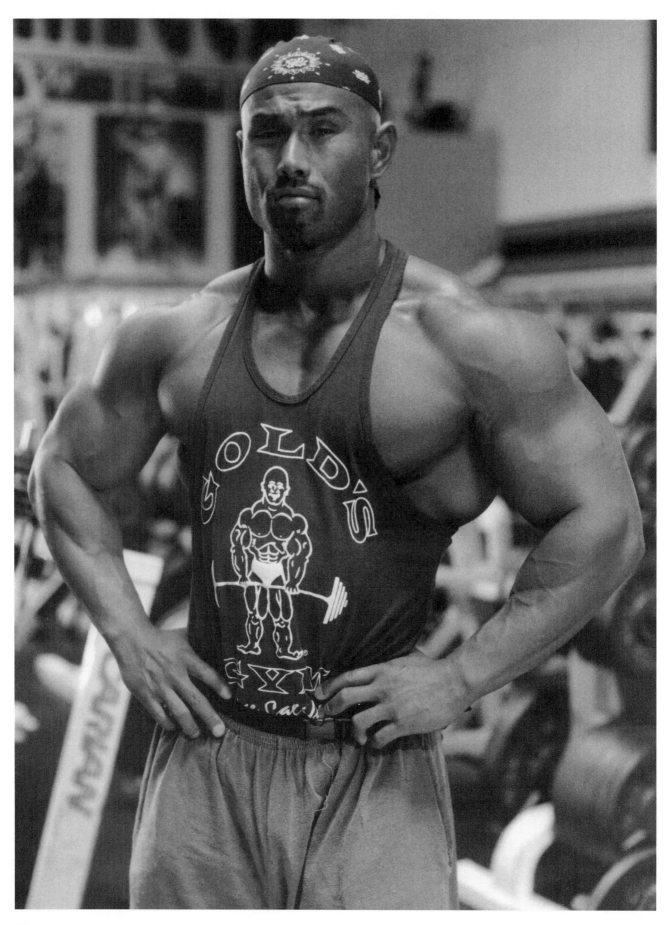

What are you guys trying to prove?

What Are You Guys Trying to Prove?

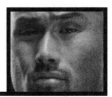

Arthur Stanley Eddington (1882–1944) was a brilliant English astronomer whose work was instrumental in proving, mathematically and experimentally, Einstein's theory of relativity. Eddington is also remembered for using an analogy to explain a complex problem involving sensory perception and scientific inquiry. He compared a fishing net to the human senses and to the parameters of any experiment. If the net has holes of a certain size, we can predict what size fish it will catch, but we cannot assume that the net will catch everything in the ocean. Hence, differently designed nets will catch different objects. Human senses have the same limitations as the fishing net, and so do experiments.

With this in mind, when we set up our Static Contraction Research Study (SCRS), we wanted to know its "bottom line" benefits for bodybuilders. We designed the first experiment to determine and measure specific factors that are important to bodybuilders:

- Would a static hold cause an increase in muscle mass?
- Would it cause a reduction in body fat?
- Would it cause an increase in muscle size?

- Would it cause an increase in both static and dynamic (full-range) strength?

We refer to these as "bottom line" benefits to distinguish them from other factors that are commonly measured in strength-training studies (what few studies there are). Frequently, for instance, parameters such as blood gases, blood chemistry, muscle fiber activity and chemistry, and electrical impulse variations are the focus of studies. Make no mistake—these are important scientific questions and are very useful measurements to know, but in the final analysis they don't really matter to bodybuilders. A bodybuilder works up a sweat to get bigger biceps, not to enjoy faster nerve discharges from his brain. Bodybuilders ultimately care about the elements we wanted to determine in the SCRS. Increased neuroelectrical stimulation of a muscle due to lifting a five-pound weight is indeed interesting, but does it put more mass on you? Does it increase the size of your biceps? Does it increase your bench press? Ultimately, these are the principal factors bodybuilders are concerned with, so we designed our "net" to find these answers.

DESIGNING THE SCRS

We recruited test subjects directly from our customer list. A small percentage of our best customers (those who had purchased multiple products over time and thus appeared to be serious bodybuilders) were asked if they would volunteer to participate in a research study involving 10 weeks of Static Contraction Training. They were asked to abandon all other forms of strength training but to make no changes in their diet, supplementation (if any), or aerobic exercise schedules. Subjects who took growth drugs of any kind were not permitted to participate. At the beginning of the study, the following data were recorded for each subject: age; weight; body fat percentage; and measurements of chest, waist, shoulders, biceps, forearm, wrist, thigh, and calf. Also, each subject was asked to characterize his own muscular development on a scale of 1 to 10 (1 representing "terrible muscular condition, very weak" and 10 representing "top of your genetic muscular limit, could not be stronger").

Next, three measurements of strength were taken:

- A conventional full-range 1-rep maximum (1RM)
- A conventional full-range 10-rep maximum (10RM)
- A static hold, in the strongest range—the range of motion where the most weight can be held—of the maximum weight possible for 15 seconds (A weight sufficiently heavy that, after 15 seconds, it could no longer be held statically and thus began to descend.)

These three measurements were taken in the following exercises: deadlift, weighted crunch, bench press, barbell shrug, lat pulldown, close-grip bench

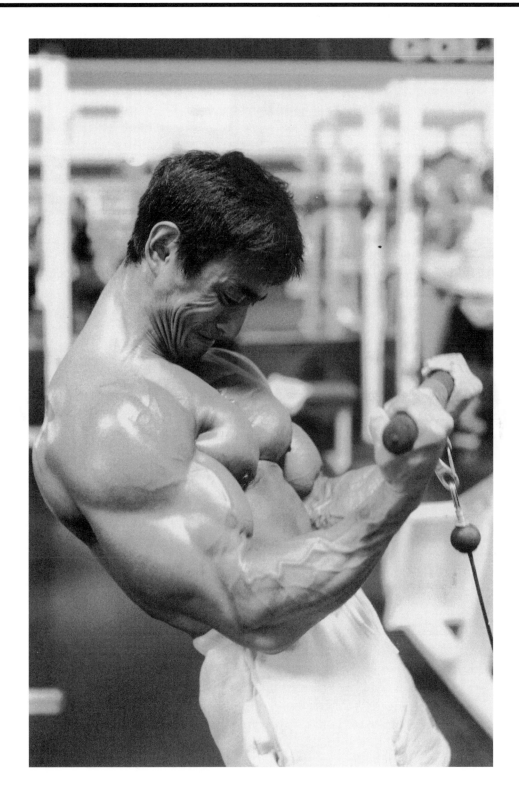

press, preacher curl, squat, leg press, calf raise, toe press, cable row, cable push-down, standing barbell curl, leg extension, and leg curl. It should be noted that because of equipment limitations, some subjects could not perform all of these exercises. However, all the exercises they did measure were still compared in before-and-after tests on the same equipment. After 10 weeks, all of the mass, size, and strength measurements were taken again for the purposes of comparison.

The workouts were divided into three major protocols involving (a) one set, (b) two sets, and (c) three sets of repetitions. Note that the term *repetitions* does not have its conventional meaning here as there is no actual movement of the weight in Static Contraction Training. In this study, a repetition consisted of holding the weight slightly out of the locked position (in the strongest range) for a period not less than 15 seconds but not more than 30 seconds.

Also, training frequencies were divided into groups of (a) three times per week, (b) two times per week and, (c) a variable schedule that began as three times per week but decreased as the study progressed.

All subjects performed workouts that consisted of a total of 10 compound exercises divided into two separate workouts of five exercises each. The first five exercises were performed on one training day, and the other five exercises were performed on the next training day. Thus, it took two different workouts in order to exercise all major muscle groups.

A *static hold* for each exercise was performed in the following manner: using the bench press as an example, the weight was moved from a resting point at the top of the subject's reach, lowered from the point of "lockout" to two or three inches below lockout (strongest range), and held there without any up or down motion.

The duration of sets performed was as follows:

1. A beginning weight was selected that could be held statically for a period of only 15 seconds. After 15 seconds the weight would begin to descend (or ascend, in the case of a lat pulldown or similar pulling movement).

2. Intensity was increased by progressively holding the weight for longer periods of time (for example, 21 seconds, 26 seconds, and so on). When a weight could be held for 30 seconds, the weight was then increased sufficiently so that the subject could hold the weight for only 15 seconds, and the progression (with the new weight) would start over. For example, a subject who could hold 100 pounds statically for 15 seconds would, on his next workout, try to hold it a little longer. In the next workout, the subject would use the same weight but try to hold it for even longer. As soon as he was up to 30 seconds with the 100-pound weight, he would increase the weight to, say, 125 pounds so that he was again able to hold it statically for only 15 seconds.

Please note that this means that the five exercises in a workout are performed with a total exercise time of 75 seconds to 2½ minutes (assuming one set per exercise). That's only 2½ minutes for the entire workout! Of course, as a practical matter, additional time is spent setting up equipment and resting between sets. While this is an extremely brief duration of maximum muscular contraction, the intensity is proportionately enormously high and has to be experienced to be fully appreciated.

As you will soon discover in the pages of this book, the results of this study were truly amazing. The universal size and strength increases, the short exercise time, and the fact that the exercises involved zero range of motion or movement indicated to us that this was something truly revolutionary.

We organized another study to measure the effects of a still greater reduction of static hold time, the number of exercise "sets," and frequency of training. This study corroborated the first and has led to more research, all of which will be revealed in the following pages. This is the first time in strength-training history that bodybuilders have had this revolutionary information, which has the power to change forever how people will train with maximum efficiency to build muscle size and strength.

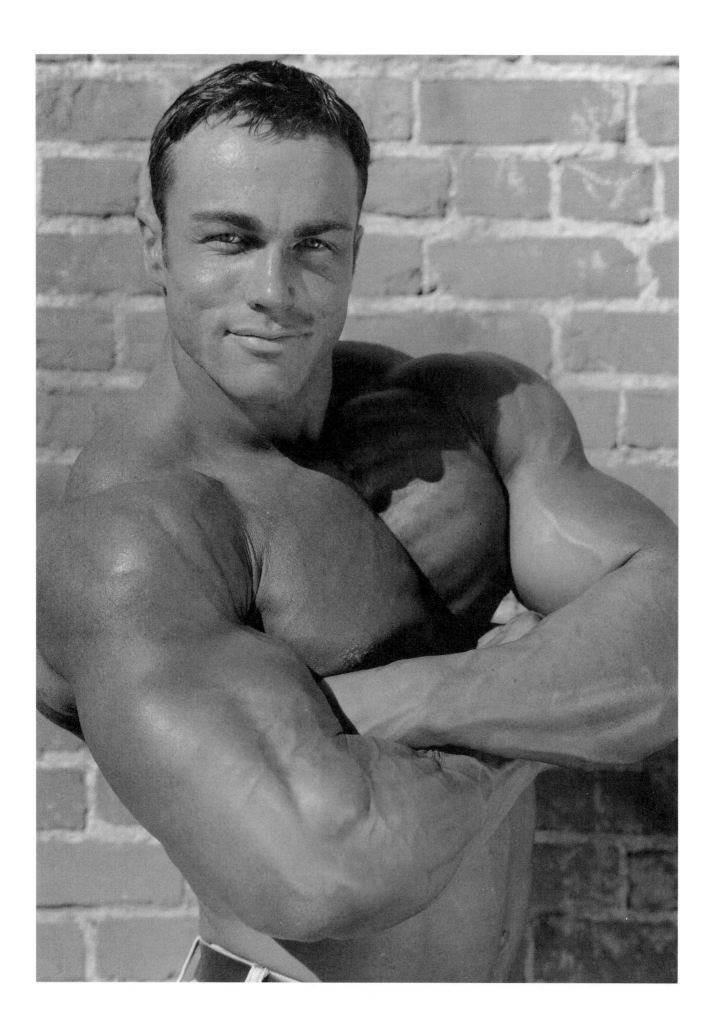

2

Why Static Contractions?

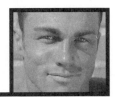

Perhaps you're wondering why we were so interested in testing static contractions as a means of increasing muscle mass and strength in the first place. Well, there were at least three reasons.

First, John developed a curiosity for the method during, of all things, a college lecture on logic. If the maximum number of muscle fibers are contracted when in the range of maximal contraction with a maximum weight, he thought, then why not force them to perform only when maximally contracted with the heaviest weight possible? What is the benefit of operating muscles under minimal or nominal contraction when it is easily possible to operate them exclusively in the maximally contracted position?

This led John to investigate what research had been done on the subject. He found existing research so fascinating, yet virtually unknown to most bodybuilders, that it became the second reason for looking further. John did some research on his own but never published his results.

Finally, when we introduced our Power Factor Training strength-training program in 1993, we recommended that all exercises be performed in only the strongest range so as to maximize muscular overload. The technique was amazingly effective and has been adopted by at least 30,000 bodybuilders worldwide. However, from that huge pool of subjects we quickly learned that many people

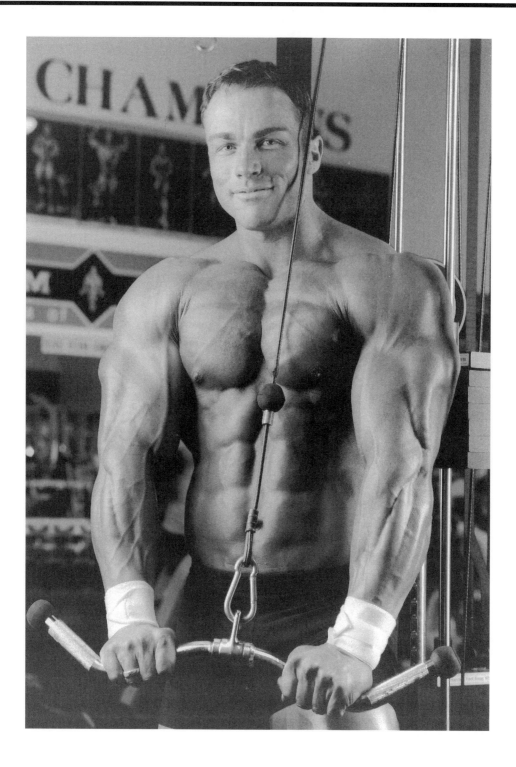

performing strong-range partials had reduced their range of motion to 50 percent or less of what we had recommended! These people claimed to be getting some of the best results of their lives. We began to wonder: How small can the effective range of motion be? Could it be zero? Our curiosity could wait no more, so we designed the SCRS to find out for ourselves.

Before we examine the results of the SCRS, it is important to understand the fundamentals that underlie its development and relate to bodybuilding principles in general. Without a basic understanding of these fundamentals, you would be taking what we recommend with a great measure of faith; that will do none of us a service. The rest of this chapter will cover the fundamentals in detail.

MUSCLE GROWTH: A SLOW PROCESS

The first step in acquiring a realistic view of building larger muscles is accepting the fact that gains in muscular mass—at least those derived from honest training—are not always rapidly forthcoming. In fact, in many cases dietary indiscretions and training errors are the direct result of bodybuilders' failure to realize just how slow the growth process truly is. After months of no progress, bodybuilders often become (if they weren't already) irrational and begin training more often, utilizing different set/rep combinations, varying hand spacing, using more free weights, or increasing protein or supplement intake. These are all things that the muscle magazines tell them to do to overcome the "inevitable" plateaus and gain those muscular pounds. They, and you, can avoid all of this frustration.

Just how slow is the growth process? Well, most exercise physiologists and seasoned bodybuilders agree that gaining even 10 pounds of muscle a year is a considerable achievement. Not 10 pounds of body weight (fat)—that's easy—but 10 pounds of pure muscle. Admittedly, 10 pounds of muscle doesn't sound like much beef, and in all candor it's not sufficient mass to alter one's appearance markedly. But over the longer term—say five years, which is how you have to look at your bodybuilding career—gaining at that rate of speed you would have packed on 50 pounds of rock-solid muscle. Now that certainly represents a considerable change in your appearance, doesn't it? In fact, it's enough to transform the average adult male weighing 165 pounds into a 215-pound Mr. Olympia competitor!

Let's assume that you can gain 10 pounds of muscle a year. Granted, we don't always think in terms of years; we think about daily progress. And with this in mind, we step on the scale every day to see whether we're "packing on the beef." What will I weigh today? we ask, as if 24 hours is ample time for any one of us to suddenly metamorphose into Arnold Schwarzenegger. But let's hold fast to our first rule—muscle growth is a slow process. When viewed in this more realistic light, we learn that growth is almost imperceptible on a daily level. Think about it. If you divide the projected muscle gain of 10 pounds by the amount of days it's going to take to gain it (365 days, or one year), you see that the number works out to .027 pounds of muscle gained per day. This is the same as 12 grams, or less than half an ounce. In fact, it's not even enough weight to register on a scale! Yet how many of us continue to weigh ourselves every day, looking for some kind of weight gain?

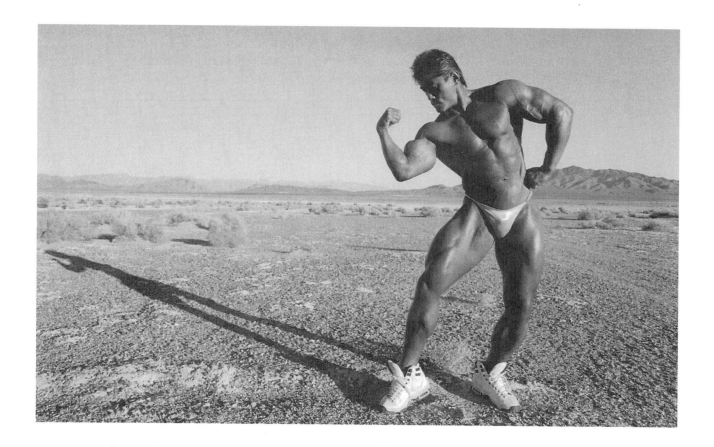

THE ROLE OF GENETICS

The second principle you need to understand in order to develop a realistic perspective on the subject of muscle building is the matter of genetics. Let it be understood that the champion bodybuilders of yesterday, today, and tomorrow are all massively muscled primarily because of one quality—exceptionally good genes. There can be no downplaying the importance of heredity in laying the foundations for a championship physique. It's hard to place a percentage figure on the role of genetics or to attempt to quantify it, but were we to do so the figure would be close to 75 percent.

Although the physiological principles involved in stimulating muscle growth are universal, certain genetic factors modify an individual's response to such stimulation. Age and sex, for example, while important, are not the predominant indices of physical superiority. Aside from the psychological traits necessary to pursue any goal to its fulfillment, a plethora of genetic factors is by far the most important consideration in your quest to develop a championship physique. Although anyone can improve upon existing levels of physical development with proper training and nutrition, only those with an abundance of the required genetic traits will become champions. These traits are skeletal formation, muscle fiber density, muscle belly length, metabolism, and physical proportions.

Skeletal Formation

Perhaps the most important genetic trait is skeletal formation. The size and formation of an individual's bones dictate how much muscle can be supported, as well as such aesthetic factors as taper and sweep that collectively make up the aesthetic quality of the physique. For instance, an individual with a bone structure like that of Bruce Lee could never develop or support the musculature of Lou Ferrigno. Conversely, an individual such as former Olympic weightlifting champion Paul Anderson could never acquire the aesthetic flow and taper of Lee. The champion bodybuilder, then, usually has a skeleton that merges these two extremes.

Muscle Fiber Density

A genetic trait that is not so readily apparent is muscle fiber density, defined as the number of fibers packed within a given volume of muscle. A person whose biceps have one-third the number of fibers of his training partner's will appear to have smaller biceps, even if he doubles their size while his partner's remain the same (provided, of course, that his biceps were proportionately smaller to begin with).

Muscle Belly Length

Interestingly, while the size of one's skeleton enables an individual to support massive muscles with great contractile power, the ultimate size a muscle might develop is dictated primarily by its length. The longer a muscle, the greater its potential for acquiring extra mass. The length of the bone to which the muscle is attached is of no great importance—it is the length from the point where the tendon attaches to the muscle at one end to the point where the tendon attaches to that muscle at the other end that determines how much size a muscle will appear to have.

Metabolism

Not everyone has the metabolic capability that allows for the creation of larger-than-normal muscle mass. We've all witnessed the efforts of the zealot who trains harder than everyone else, yet never shows any visible signs of improvement. If you have been training smart and hard for a couple of years, and have made only very minimal gains in muscular mass, you're probably not geared metabolically for the development of large muscles. Many, however, could gain more quickly than their present rate of growth might indicate if they were to adopt a proper training program.

Physical Proportions

Superior athletes in any sport possess physical proportions ideally suited to their sport. Sprinters, for example, usually have short torsos, narrow hips, and long legs. The ideal proportions of a middle linebacker are a long torso, short legs, wide hips, and long arms. Bodybuilders require balanced proportions since their "sport" is more aesthetic. However, even those select few, the "thoroughbreds" who do possess a superabundance of the required traits, will

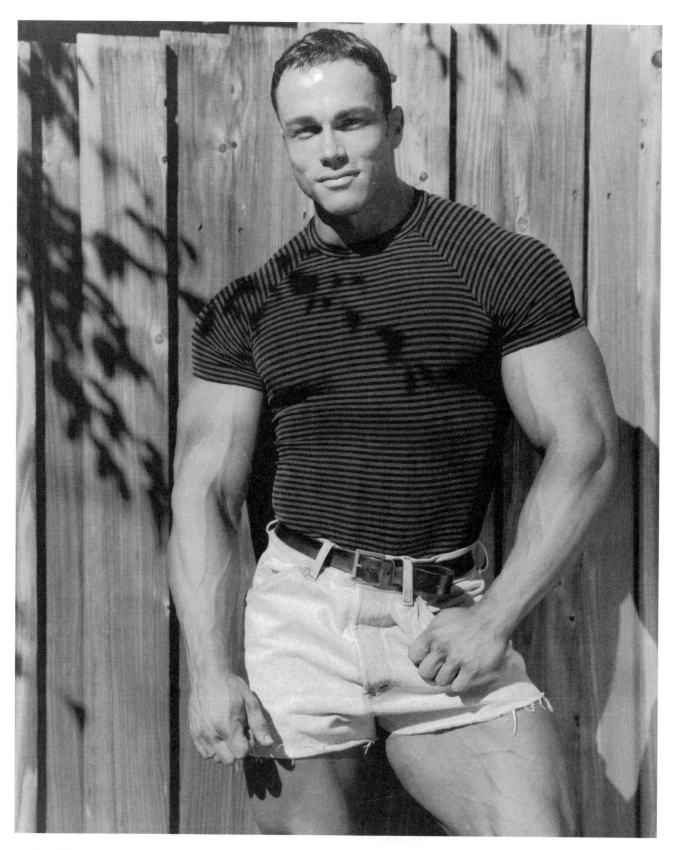

Look at the length of the unflexed biceps! That's a purely genetic trait that cannot be changed.

improve more quickly and go much farther if they train and diet intelligently. The reason is that while these variances in genetic endowment are the ultimate indices of future bodybuilding success, the physiology underlying both the genetically gifted and the merely average person are universal and apply equally to all human beings.

THE PROBLEM WITH TRADITION

While this may sound shocking to many of you, the training routines of most of our "Mr." titleists (Mr. Universe, Mr. Olympia, Mr. World, and so on) are next to useless. Having worked alongside all of the top champions in the field for over 12 years, we can assure you that most of them operate on a hit-or-miss basis, often mistaking muscle soreness for stimulation and inefficient training methods for productive ones. Further, they typically eat like pigs to bulk up and then eat like birds to trim down; and eventually they consume huge quantities of anabolic steroids, human growth hormone (HGH), and diuretics to aid them in doing both (a further testament to the inefficacy of their training routines).

Ignorance, it would seem, springs eternal, and this is why still today confusion abounds regarding how to train correctly for maximum increases in muscle mass. Few, it seems, are willing to apply the foolproof method of logic and rationality to their search for the ideal training routine. Few are willing to spend time engaged in the one activity that would actually aid them in their search for a more productive way to train—the activity of productive, rational thought.

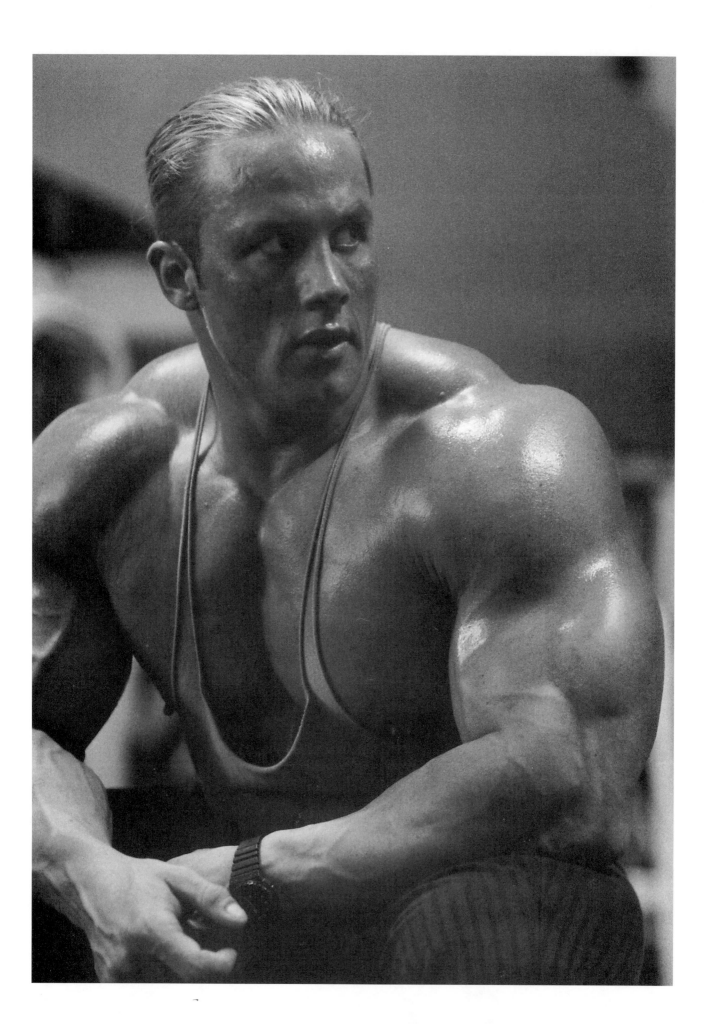

3

Progress and Overtraining

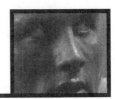

If you follow the guidelines of this program to the letter, you will experience an absolute minimum of overtraining. We cannot say *zero* overtraining because the frequency of workouts actually remains fixed until the first sign of overtraining. For example, you might train once per week for nine weeks with steady progress, but on the tenth week notice that your numbers did not improve. That, in the simplest terms, means that you just engaged in overtraining. This will be immediately apparent when you record your numbers on your training log. When overtraining occurs, you simply need to space your workouts farther apart. If you stubbornly continue to train on a too-frequent basis, you will develop a number of telltale symptoms. The most common are an almost constant sense of fatigue combined with a deep lack of energy and ambition. Other signs include:

- Frequent colds and injuries
- Persistent soreness and stiffness in the muscles, joints, or tendons
- Feeling of heaviness in your legs
- Loss of interest in training
- Inability to relax
- Decrease in academic work or performance

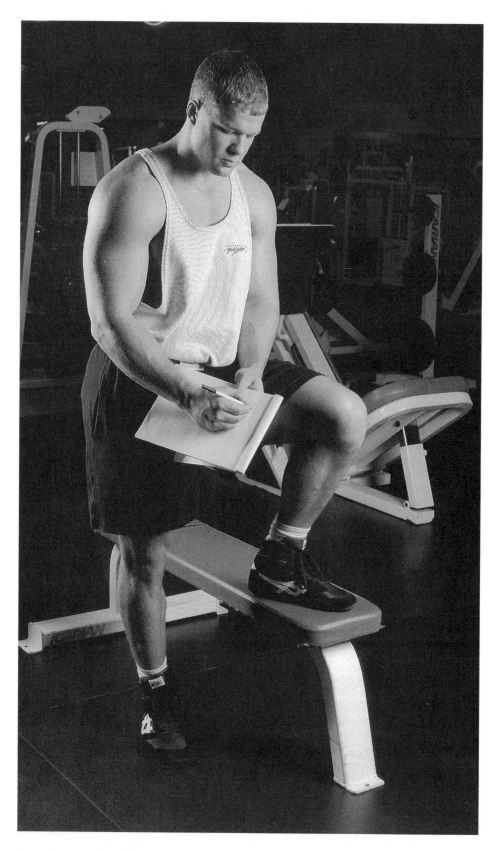

A log of your weights and times is critical for keeping track of what is working and what is not.

- Sleep problems
- Headaches
- Loss of appetite

One of the more popular methods used to detect overtraining is to monitor the morning pulse rate. Upon arising, take your pulse for 60 seconds. If it is seven beats a minute faster than usual, a layoff or reduction in training is indicated. Perhaps the most blatant symptom of overtraining is a very strong disinclination to train at all, as your body is signaling your brain that it hasn't fully recovered from the cumulative systemic toll of previous training sessions. Any person who falls into the habit of training five or six days a week over a prolonged period of time will inevitably become overtrained, regardless of how powerful or well built he may be.

THE NECESSITY OF A TRAINING LOG

As there are many exercises, weights, and hold times to be remembered in Static Contraction Training, it's exceedingly difficult to retain all of the knowledge you have gathered. Steady progress can only be ensured by using a log to record the specifics of each workout.

Our sample training log (see below) shows how this form is used. Notice how the weights and times show progression in successive workouts. The

Workout A							
	Zero	One	Three	Five	Seven	Nine	Eleven
Exercise	Date: *Aug 1*	Date: *Aug 15*	Date: *Sept 1*	Date: *Sept 15*	Date: *Oct 1*	Date:	Date:
Shoulder press	140/5 lbs/sec	140/13	160/9	160/17	185/5	/	/
Cable row	145/9 lbs/sec	170/6	170/13	190/5	190/17	/	/
Crunch	50/10 lbs/sec	60/5	60/14	65/5	65/9	/	/
Bench press	210/8 lbs/sec	210/19	240/6	240/15	270/10	/	/
Shrug	290/10 lbs/sec	305/8	305/20	350/8	370/8	/	/
Wrist curl	40/10 lbs/sec	50/10	50/17	65/8	65/16	/	/

This is a sample training log for Workout A. Notice the progression of both weights and hold times. Also note that an extra exercise was included for this subject.

Workout A							
	Zero	**One**	**Three**	**Five**	**Seven**	**Nine**	**Eleven**
Exercise	Date:	Date:	Date:	Date:	Date:	Date:	Date:
	/	/	/	/	/	/	/
	/	/	/	/	/	/	/
	/	/	/	/	/	/	/
	/	/	/	/	/	/	/
	/	/	/	/	/	/	/
	/	/	/	/	/	/	/

Photocopy this blank form for record keeping.

Workout B							
	Zero	**Two**	**Four**	**Six**	**Eight**	**Ten**	**Twelve**
Exercise	Date:	Date:	Date:	Date:	Date:	Date:	Date:
	/	/	/	/	/	/	/
	/	/	/	/	/	/	/
	/	/	/	/	/	/	/
	/	/	/	/	/	/	/
	/	/	/	/	/	/	/
	/	/	/	/	/	/	/

Photocopy this blank form for record keeping.

blank log forms (see page 18) may be photocopied for your own use. You will notice that Workout A contains odd numbers and Workout B contains even numbers to ensure that the workouts are done alternately. When you complete Workouts 11 and 12, enter new numbers under Workout Zero on new A and B log forms and continue training. We cannot overstate the importance of using logs for success with this program.

THE ROLE OF INTENSITY

The key to bodybuilding success is concentrated bursts of very high-intensity muscular contraction: the higher the intensity, the greater the growth stimulation. Intensity and duration exist in an inverse ratio to one another; in other words, you can train hard (intensity) or you can train long (duration), but you can't do both. The fact of the matter is that it takes hard—*brutally hard*—training to develop massive muscles if you intend to do so without the artificial aid of growth-enhancing drugs, and this system is the hardest in which you will ever engage. As a result, Static Contraction Training will prove to be the most productive method of bodybuilding you'll ever experience.

Intensity is a widely misunderstood concept, at least as it applies to muscle building. When applied to bodybuilding, and more specifically to one's training efforts to build the body, intensity is simply one of two possible components of any exercise session, the second component being duration. Duration is the length of any given training session, whereas intensity describes the degree of effort put forth during the session. The problem arises when people confuse the two terms, thinking that by increasing the duration of their workouts they somehow increase intensity. This just isn't true.

The fact is that just the opposite is true; when you increase the duration of an exercise session by adding either sets or reps to the routine, you must decrease the intensity of your training to allow for the additional energy expenditure. These two components exist in an inverse ratio to one another and, consequently, are mutually exclusive. That is to say, you can't have one and the other existing to the same degree or in the same capacity in the same space and time.

This inverse ratio has been graphed by exercise physiologists to demonstrate the universal relationship (see graph on page 21). The bipolar relationship between intensity and duration is both immutable and universal and, consequently, is one of the more basic laws of physics. It applies to all activities, from concentration to weight training. The more intensely you do something, the more you must decrease the duration of that activity. And if you want to build big muscles as quickly as possible, you've got to train as intensely as possible because that is the prime requisite in the stimulation of muscle growth. In other words, if you want to build muscular mass, you've got to train for short periods of time so that you'll be able to train intensely. That, in essence, is the nature of the relationship: you can either train hard or you can train long—but you can't do both.

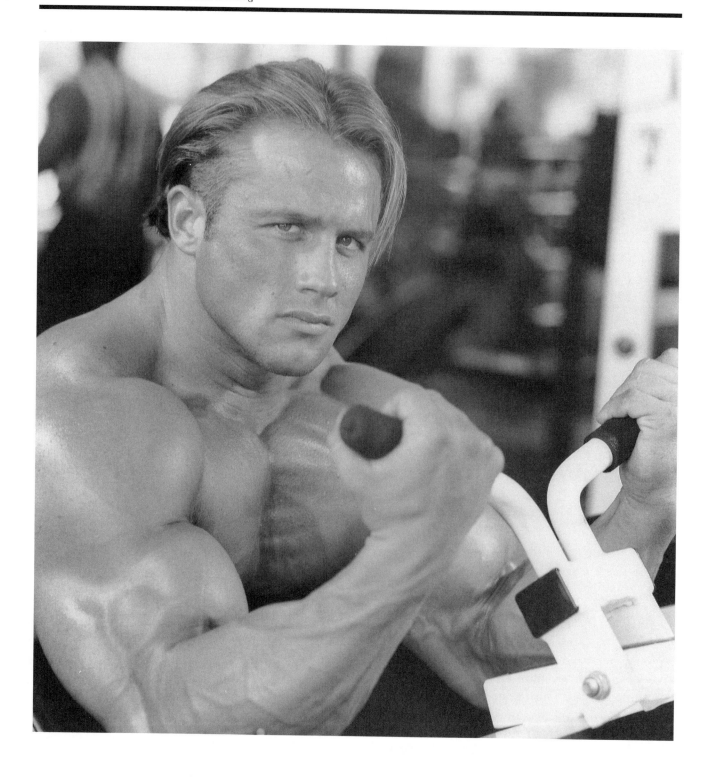

For example, no one, no matter how fit, can engage in an all-out sprint for a mile. Why? Because an all-out sprint is a maximum-intensity activity and therefore cannot be engaged in for any appreciable distance over 400 meters. Consequently, anyone who tells you that he's training "intensely" for a period of time that stretches beyond a few minutes (and some bodybuilders will "train" in the gym for up to three hours) is displaying a profound ignorance of this basic principle of physics.

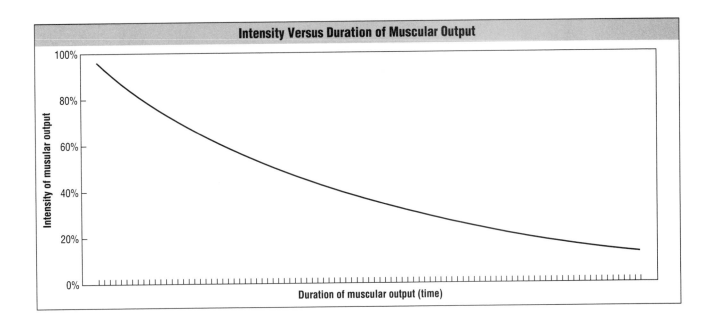

The bodybuilders you read about who train for hours at a time are more like distance runners than sprinters. For the most part, they chronically overtrain and would probably look more like their distance-running counterparts were it not for the massive amount of anabolic steroids (and other growth-enhancing drugs) they consume that have a muscle-spurring effect. It must always be remembered that training has a negative effect on the body, as it always cuts into the body's recovery ability. And the longer you train, the more recovery ability you use up. Like the distance runner, if you engage in this activity for prolonged periods of time and don't allow your recuperative subsystems time to recover, you'll not only feel overtrained, but you'll also never experience the muscular progress that you could have enjoyed had you trained properly.

Remember, you must first stimulate growth and then allow enough time for recovery to take place so that growth can ultimately occur. Your progress will be continual if you remember to do these three things:

1. Stimulate growth.
2. Allow enough time for recovery to take place.
3. Allow another period of time for the growth you have stimulated to manifest.

Growth never precedes recovery—recovery always precedes growth. It couldn't be otherwise. If you didn't continually recover from exercise you would eventually die. Obviously, if you train before recovery has occurred, the growth process can't take place. And if you allow enough time for recovery to take place but not enough time for growth to occur, you still won't grow! Why? Because it takes time for the growth process to be switched on. No one is exempt from this basic law of biology—not you, not me, not Arnold Schwarzenegger. It's not unlike the process of hair growth; it's a biological

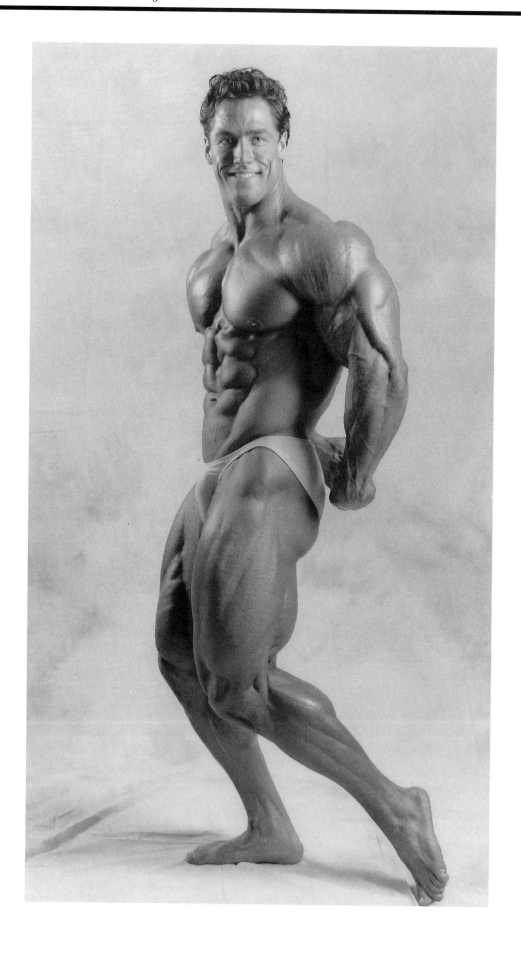

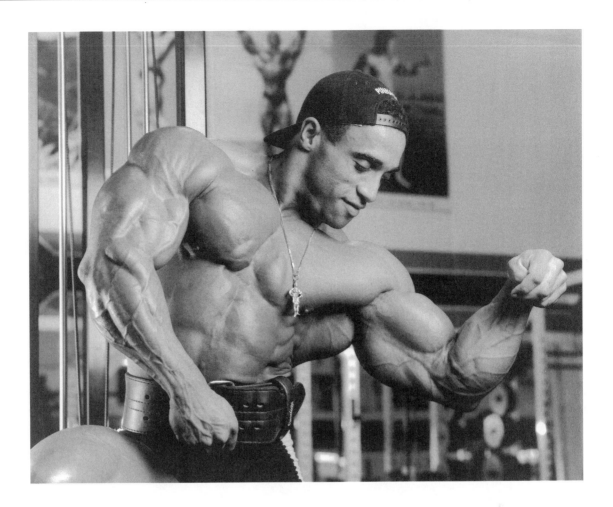

process that cannot be rushed. You could go into a hair salon every day and have your hair professionally washed, styled, and cut—but that won't in any way hasten the growth process, which, being biological in nature, cannot be affected by anything other than your DNA.

To better illustrate this point, imagine that you do as many total failure sets of heavy squats as you can on Monday. The muscles in your legs might feel fully recovered by Tuesday, so you attempt a high-intensity back training session that day. You'll find that you simply do not possess the inclination or ability to progress. The reason for this is that your whole system had been called upon for the purpose of adaptation and overcompensation the day before, when you performed the squats. Demands were made upon all of your body's recuperative subsystems, not just your legs. This is an important point to bear in mind.

Of course, if you train with low intensity, you might well be able to recover sufficiently to train again the next day, but your progress in terms of muscle mass gains will be nil. And your objective in bodybuilding should never be to see how much exercise you can tolerate, but rather just how little exercise is required to stimulate maximum increases in muscle size and strength—which is solely a product of training intensity.

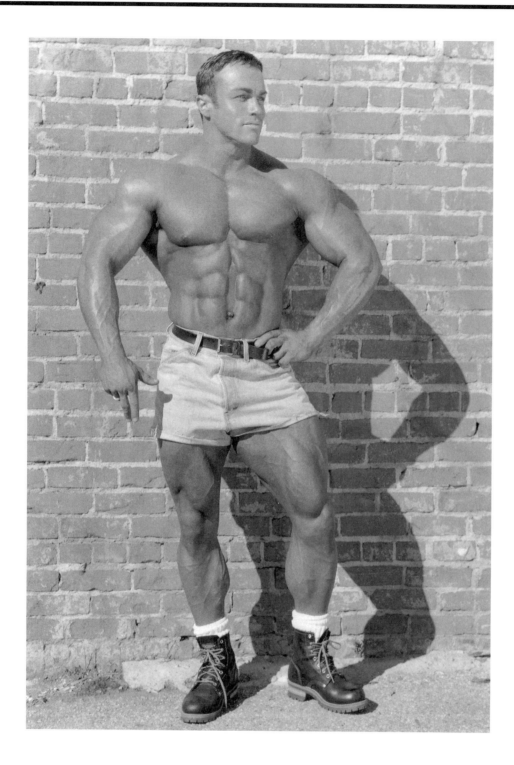

MUSCLE GROWTH—NOT AN EASY PROCESS

Nobody has yet successfully challenged the paradigm that muscle growth does not come easily—you have to force growth to occur. And you cannot force growth by contracting your muscles against light weights or performing tasks that are already well within the muscles' existing capacities. Some people have been quoted in the muscle magazines as saying that high-intensity training only works for a select few, and that if you have the genetic makeup of a super-man and take steroids, then you make do with such a system of training. Such statements only serve to reveal ignorance of high-intensity training principles and expose unwillingness to look seriously and objectively into training methodology and the science that underpins it. If a method works, it works. Period. It can't work sometimes and not work other times (given the same conditions and context). High-intensity training has the backing of exercise science to support it and consequently can be presented in a logical fashion (that is, its conclusions follow from its premises). Unfortunately, the same cannot be said for the proponents of contrary training methods. Facts cannot be ignored if verifiable knowledge and noncontradictory conclusions hold any meaning for you.

We are now aware of the supreme importance of intensity of effort, and we know that the greater the intensity applied during training, the greater the growth stimulation and the briefer the workout. What is the method that will generate maximum intensity and hence the greatest degree of muscle growth? The answer, as we shall see, awaits us in the data from our Static Contraction Research Study.

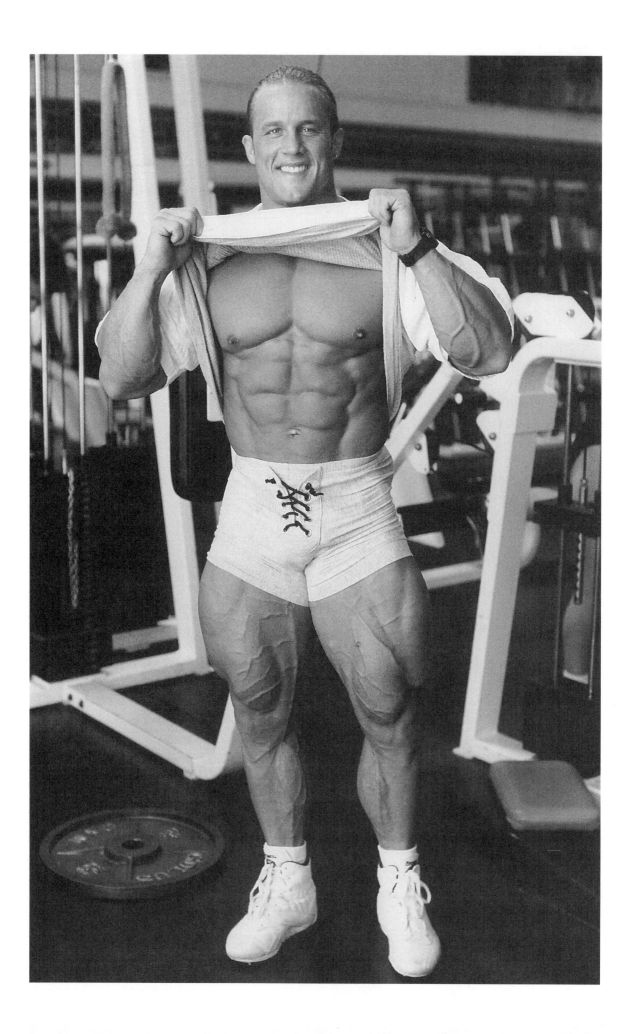

4

Muscle Building—a Look Inside

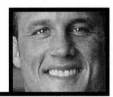

There are three distinct types of muscle within the human body. One is *cardiac* muscle, which is responsible for the contractions of your heart—not unlike the contraction of any one of the 600 discernible muscles throughout the body. One of the microscopic differences that separates cardiac muscle from skeletal muscle is the existence of physiological "generators" on certain cardiac muscle cells called pacemaker cells. These cells send out signals to the heart that enable it to contract. As their name implies, the function of these cells has given rise to the concept of the pacemaker, the device worn by people with certain heart conditions. The second general type of muscle, known either as *smooth* or *visceral*, lines the walls of the internal organs (the viscera) and assists in the transportation of food and waste materials to their proper destinations. The third type of muscle, the one bodybuilders are most concerned with, is *skeletal* muscle. These, of course, are the muscles of the body that are responsible for all of the movements we engage in on a daily basis. Skeletal muscles are attached from one bone to another across one or more joints. Their shortening, or contraction, is what allows us to move.

CONTRACTION

As already indicated, skeletal muscle has only one function: to shorten, or contract. This being the case, it immediately becomes apparent that training routines such as the "push/pull system" (wherein supposedly all of your "pushing muscles" are trained on one day and all of your "pulling muscles" the next) are misnomers of the highest order. The function of skeletal muscle has nothing to do with either of these two things.

The proteins, the molecular components that make up muscle fiber, cannot push outward any more than a moose can fly—it's simply not in either's physiological makeup. And yet, having said this, it would appear—if only superficially—that we can push things away from us by using our muscles. After all, we perform push-ups and push open doors. If the term doesn't exist in the realm of physiology, it's certainly alive and well in the world of popular phraseology.

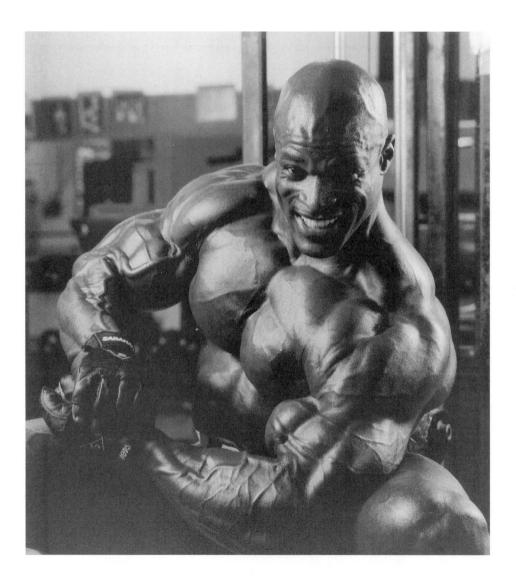

But what actually happens when we push something? Simply the activation of an antagonistic group of muscle fibers. All muscles are paired on opposite sides of a bone or a limb. There is no anatomical exception to this rule; all muscles appear in pairs (this is a corollary of the "every action has an equal and opposite reaction" law). For example, your quadriceps are paired with your

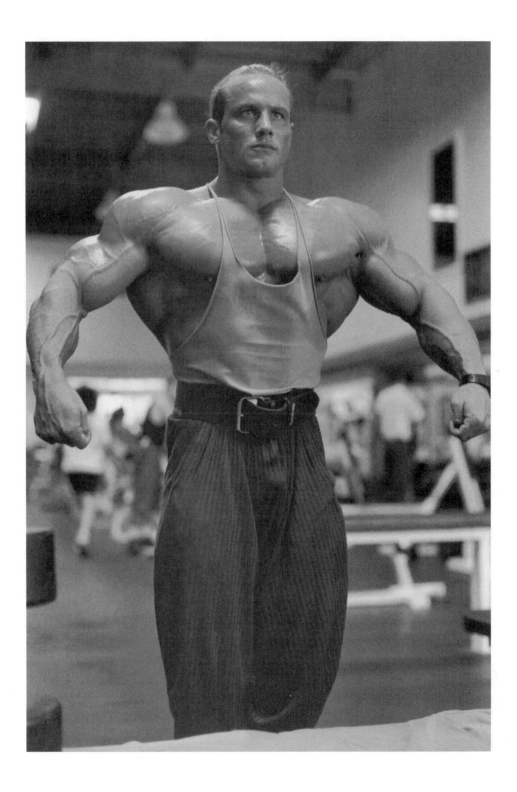

hamstrings; your forearm flexors are paired with your extensors; and your biceps are opposite your triceps. Here's how it works: Let's suppose you've just pushed the resistance on a leg press machine from the starting position to the fully extended position. Your hamstrings, or "leg biceps," are located on the lower surface of your femur (thigh bone) and attach to your lower leg. When they contract, they bring your heel and lower leg closer to your buttocks. Your quadriceps, located on the top surface of your femur, are also attached to your lower leg and are stretched when the hamstrings are contracted. Now, if you want to push that weight back to the starting position, you contract your quadriceps muscles. This, in turn, extends the lower leg back to the starting position while at the same time stretching your hamstrings. All in all, you get the appearance of pushing from the drawing together of muscle tissue.

THE BIG PICTURE

As we've now pointed out (in a very general way) how certain muscle groups function, it should be noted that these muscle groups are usually comprised of anywhere from two to four muscles, a form of team effort, if you will—at least as far as movement is involved. Some muscles arise from one bone in two or three different places only to join or insert into a second bone as one muscle. Now hold on, there's nothing mystical about this—it's just human physiology in action, pure and simple. Here's a sampling of some of these "team" muscles:

Hamstrings: This muscle group is composed of three muscles: the semitendinosus, the semimembranosus, and the biceps femoris. The hamstrings are situated behind the femur.

Quadriceps: This is a four-muscle composite consisting of the vastus

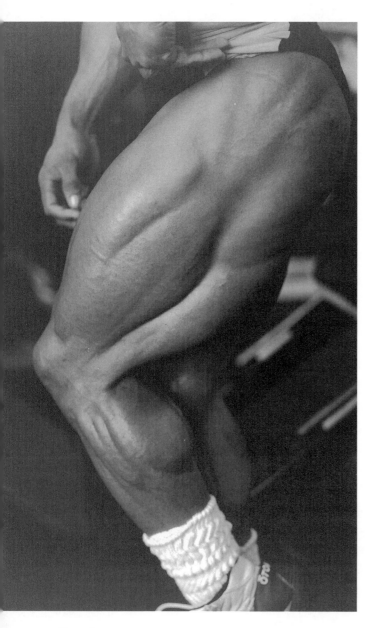

Hamstrings.

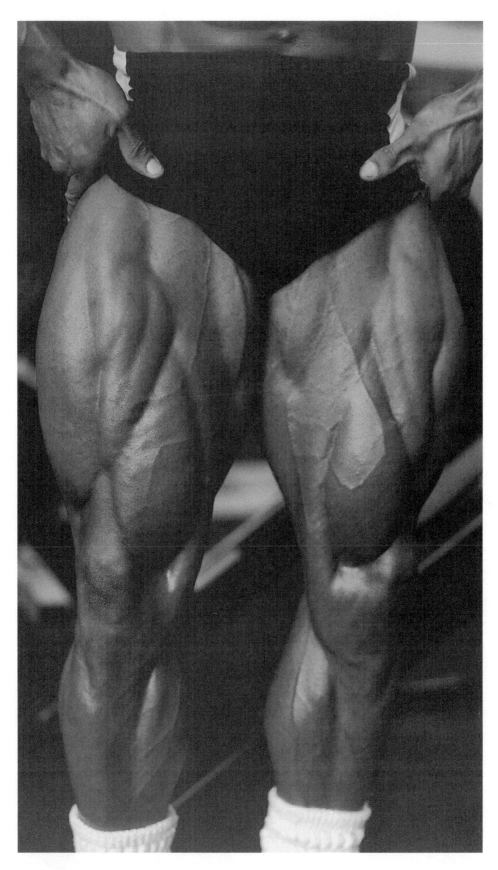

Quadriceps.

lateralis, the vastus medialis, the vastus intermedius, and the rectus femoris. All of these muscles reside on the front of the femur.

Deltoids: This is a three-muscle team that covers the entire shoulder cap. It consists of the anterior deltoid (the front head), the lateral deltoid (the side head), and the posterior deltoid (the rear head). Each head of the deltoid possesses an individual function that results in shoulder movement, and specific exercises are required to fully stimulate each head of the muscle.

Biceps: A two-headed muscle located on the front of the upper arm that originates on two points of the scapula (shoulder blade) and inserts into one point in the forearm.

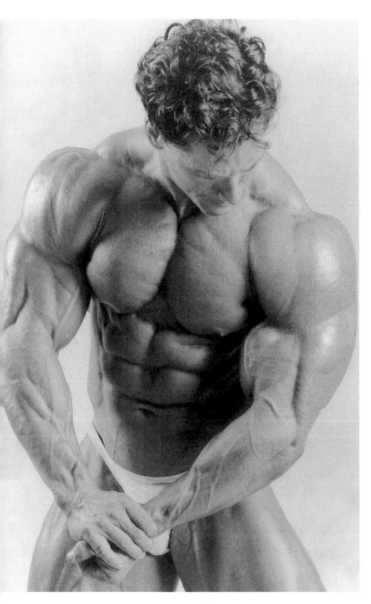

Deltoids.

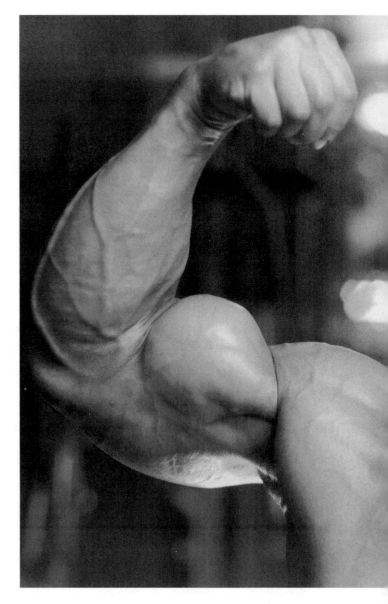

Biceps.

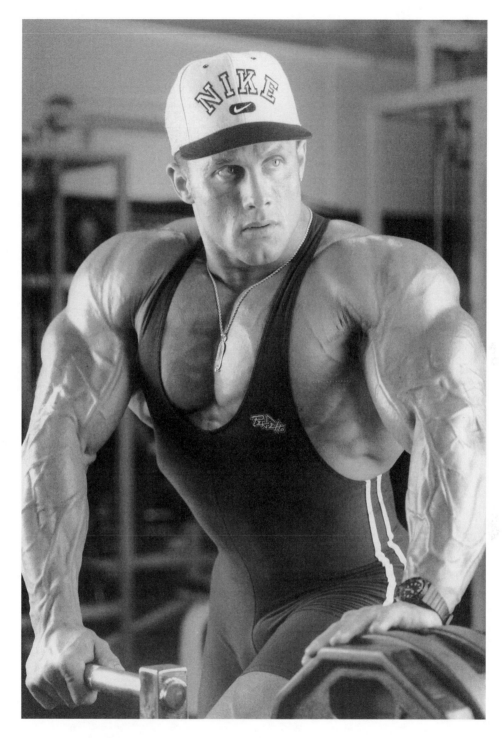

Triceps account for about two-thirds of the size of the upper arm.

Triceps: A three-headed muscle located on the rear of the upper arm with three different origins on the shoulder that come together to insert into one attachment on the forearm. Different exercises will stress (to a limited degree) different heads of the muscle.

THE SMALL PICTURE

Each muscle is composed of fibers that collectively form specific muscles. Each muscle fiber, as small as it is, is nevertheless the shell of a bundle of even smaller fibers. These smaller fibers are known as *myofibrils* and even these contain smaller fibrous components known as *myofilaments*. So, to repeat, your muscles are made up of bundles of fibers, which are made up of bundles of myofibrils, which in turn are made up of bundles of myofilaments.

Here's a staggering statistic from the world of science: the average person has been estimated to have over one quarter of a billion muscle fibers in his body. You can well appreciate the math required to calculate the total amount of myofilaments one might have! In any event, what all of these bundles have in common, from the fiber down to the myofilament, is the denominator of contraction. To this end, they enlist the aid of two of the four proteins that reside in muscle tissue, *actin* and *myosin*. Both actin and myosin are referred to as *contractile proteins* because their function is to hook up and contract, which creates muscular force or tension which is important for stimulating muscle growth. The remaining two proteins are *troponin* and *tropomyosin*, and their role is like that of an "off switch" mechanism for the actin and myosin.

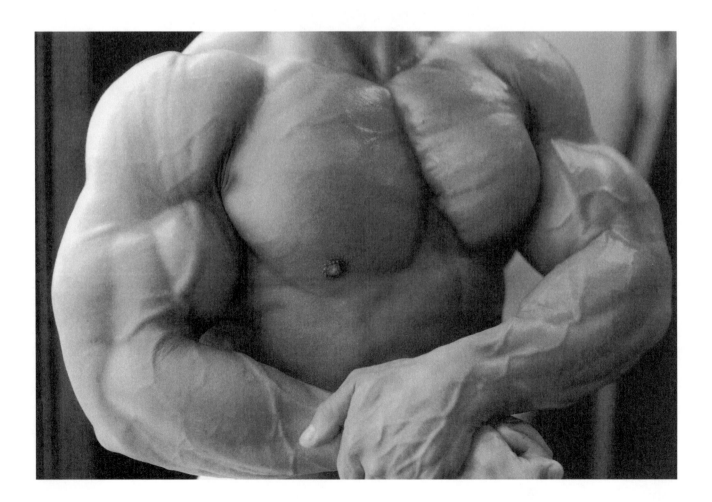

The nature of actin and myosin is that, when left unimpeded, they seek out each other and draw toward one another. Unless the other two proteins (troponin and tropomyosin) step into the equation, actin and myosin find each other and muscular contraction occurs. In fact, were it not for the wedge-like effect of troponin and tropomyosin, you would be in constant agony because your muscles would always be contracted maximally (cramping).

Having stated that proteins are a part of muscle tissue, we should point out that muscle tissue isn't all protein. Further, you don't need a lot of supplemental protein (such as pills or powders) in your diet in order to build larger muscles. The truth of the matter is that only 22 percent of a muscle is composed of protein; the remainder, more than 70 percent, is water. Believe us—you will do nothing to hasten the muscle growth process by consuming excessive amounts of protein.

The Root of Contraction

Muscle contraction begins with an electrical signal from the central nervous system. When the current arrives at the muscle, it is immediately transferred up and down the length and depth of the muscle through a relay system of tubules. When the message reaches each one of the thousands of receptor sites, it drops off a little shot of calcium. Calcium inhibits the noncontractile proteins troponin and tropomyosin, which, until the calcium showed up, had been doing their job of keeping the actin and myosin proteins separated. The calcium has the same effect on troponin and tropomyosin that kryptonite has on Superman—it takes away their power to separate actin and myosin, inhibiting their ability to function—and their function, of course, is to keep the contractile proteins from contracting.

Further analysis reveals this process even more clearly when we look at the *sarcomere*, which is simply one individual unit of actin and myosin. At each end of the sarcomere is a rather broad anchoring structure called a *z-disc*. And extending inward from each z-disc are thin strands of actin that just manage to overlap the much thicker strands of myosin that reside smack-dab in the middle of each sarcomere.

Myosin protein strands have little receptor sites that emanate outward from either side of their main bodies that resemble something of a cross between little hooks and the strands of a feather. Technically, these receptor sites are called *cross bridges*, as they serve to bridge or connect actin and myosin.

Once the electrical charge for contraction arrives via the nerve cells from the brain to the muscle, the nerve cells drop off a little packet of calcium that immediately severs the leashlike effect of the troponin and tropomyosin. With the leash removed, so to speak, several rather phenomenal actions take place involving the now free-floating actin and myosin:

- The cross bridges rotate and in so doing draw the actin filaments and z-discs inward ever so slightly.
- The cross bridges begin to attach to the actin protein strands.
- The proteins themselves undergo a change in shape.
- The sarcomere shortens as both z-discs are drawn inward.

When many of these sarcomeres shorten simultaneously, the muscle fibers—and then the muscle itself—contract. And, although some textbooks may tell you that the shortening of the sarcomere is caused by the release of energy caused by a breakdown of ATP (*adenosine triphosphate*), this is not the case. In fact, the process of contraction will occur automatically whenever calcium enters the picture, thus inhibiting the restrictive function of the troponin and tropomyosin proteins. ATP is required, however, for the cross bridges to release and return to their "resting" position until they're required to contract again. An example of this can be seen if you flex the biceps in your upper arm. This is the result of thousands of contractions and (if you extend your forearm) releases by the cross bridges, with the contracting portion precipitated by the presence of calcium and the releases fueled by the energy generated by the breakdown of ATP.

THE ROLE OF ATP

What is this ATP? Quite simply, ATP is the fundamental fuel for all bodily functions. From walking across the room to contemplating philosophical abstractions, ATP is the energy that runs the show. ATP has been described as a miniature warehouse of energy—and it is. ATP is made up of three phosphate groups: oxygen, phosphorus, and adenosine. The adenosine is really a molecule to which the oxygen and phosphorus bond to form the chemical compound adenosine triphosphate (ATP).

When energy is required for muscular contraction, ATP is the first one out of the blocks to provide it—usually by breaking off one of the phosphate groups, which leaves ADP (*adenosine diphosphate*). The result is that a good portion of energy is released for immediate use by the muscles. (ADP cannot be broken down further into AMP (*adenosine monophosphate*), by the muscles themselves; but, if needed, this can occur elsewhere in the body to create more energy for movement.)

Let's suppose you are about to begin a static contraction set and, having just come off a weeklong layoff, your energy reserves and ATP stores are completely replenished. At the start of your exercise session, you will have roughly three ounces of ATP in your entire body available to be converted to usable energy. This will be adequate to keep any muscle contracting for roughly three seconds. If your set is going to last longer than three seconds (which of course it will), you're going to need more ATP energy to successfully complete the duration of your set. So where's it going to come from? Well, the energy transporter in this case is another chemical compound called CP (*creatine phosphate*).

When CP is broken down into its molecular components of creatine and phosphate, the energy that is released can hook up with an ADP molecule and attach to it a loose phosphate molecule to create a new ATP molecule. And the neat part is that there's enough CP stored in your body to keep up this ATP conversion process for a solid 10 seconds—or the upper limits that would be required to perform a typical static contraction set.

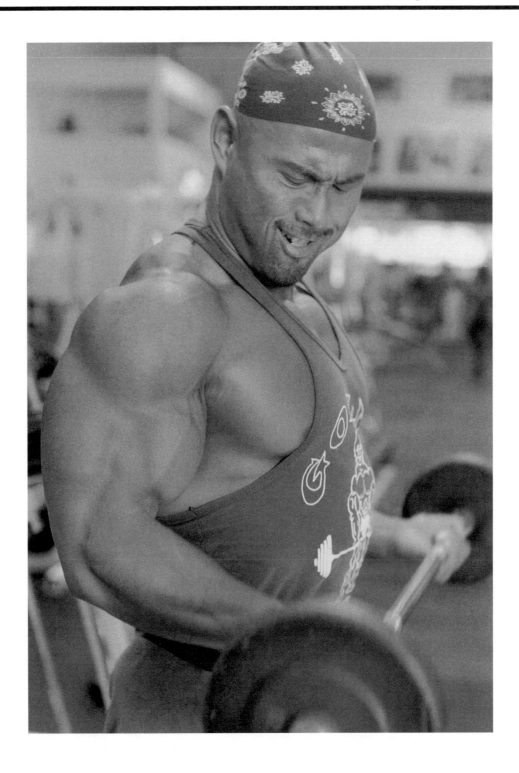

EARLY RESEARCH ON STATIC CONTRACTION

For more than 10 years, Erich A. Muller of the Max Planck Insitut für Arbeitsphysiologie experimented in Dortmund, Germany, to discover the fastest way to increase muscle strength and the essential factors necessary to produce hypertrophy. Success came when, toward the end of this period, he

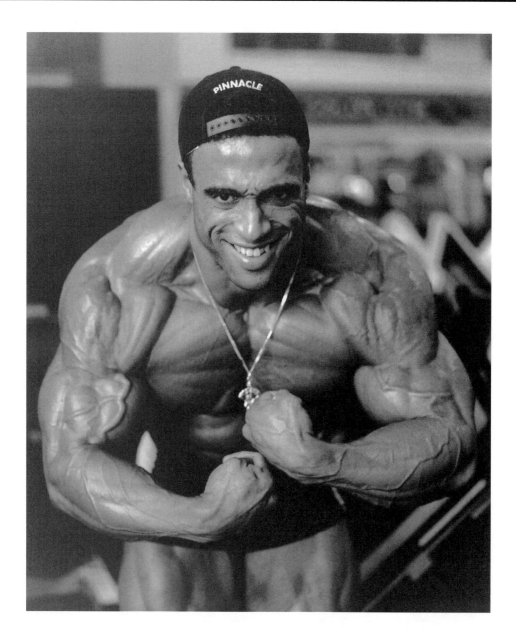

began to work with one of his students, Thomas Hettinger, on static contractions in which intensity and duration were easily measured. No less than 71 separate experiments were performed on nine male subjects over a period of 18 months.[1] All training was done in the form of pulling and holding a predetermined amount of tension against a spring scale. Most observations were made on the flexors and extensors of the forearms held horizontally at right angles to the upper arm. A number of significant findings emerged:

- Muscle strength increased an average of 5 percent per week when the training load was as little as one-third of maximal strength.
- Muscle strength increased more rapidly with increasing intensity of training load up to about two-thirds of maximal strength. *Beyond this, increase in training load had no further effect.*

- One practice period per day in which the tension was held for only six seconds resulted in as much increase in strength as longer periods (up to full exhaustion in 45 seconds) and more frequent periods (up to seven exercises per day).
- The rate of increase in strength sometimes varied considerably in the same person when two comparable training periods, separated by a long rest period, were compared.

This early research certainly corresponds with our own findings. While lighter weights will yield some benefit, heavier weights deliver greater gains at a faster rate. Also, frequent workouts are not only unnecessary; they actually serve to overtrain the body within a short period of time. Further, we have done some experimentation with hold times and have already found that reduced hold times, especially when they permit the use of heavier weights, have a beneficial, rather than deleterious, effect on both the rate and magnitude of strength gains.

THE ANAEROBIC PATHWAYS

There exist but two types of training pathways as mapped out by your central nervous system—*anaerobic* and *aerobic*. However, for the purposes of building larger, stronger muscles, you need to remain exclusively in the anaerobic pathways. Aerobic exercise mainly burns body fat for fuel and requires the presence of oxygen to do so. Aerobic training is a necessity if your objective is endurance-related activities such as distance running or cross-country skiing. However, as your objective is stimulating muscle growth and strength, you want to burn solely glycogen, which is stored within the muscles you are training, as your fuel of choice.

During the first 10 to 60 seconds of muscle contraction, energy is largely derived from your anaerobic system. With longer-duration training (wherein a typical set can run on for as long as two minutes), your body will start to employ aerobic pathways to help with the workload. In fact, after 90 to 100 seconds, the aerobic system is responsible for 50 percent of your energy output. This means, in effect, that you're splitting your training stimulus for muscle mass in half with the new request for more aerobic assistance, utilizing 50 percent of the stimulus that could have been used solely for muscle growth.

THE IMPORTANCE OF CARBOHYDRATES

It follows from this that carbohydrates, the primary fuel for muscles operating within the anaerobic pathways (since carbohydrates are readily converted to glycogen), are the nutrient of choice for the serious bodybuilder. Carbohydrates are the sole fuel for training anaerobically, which is what you want to do to stimulate increases in size and strength. Further, it takes the body up to 50 minutes of continuous exercise to begin the breakdown of fats for energy; and if carbohydrate stores in your body are low, your system will turn first to protein, which is most readily available from your lean body tissue (your muscle mass). In other words, if adequate carbohydrate isn't available for the contracting muscles through the foods you eat, the body will consume your existing stores of muscle mass for fuel! Another interesting side note for those who habitually engage in low-carbohydrate diets for the purpose of shedding body fat: people on these diets lose out on a small compound that forms as a result of the breakdown of carbohydrate into the bloodstream. This compound is essential for the metabolism of fat within the body. Beyond this, the human brain derives 99.9 percent of the nutrition it needs to survive from glucose (the form that carbohydrates take once broken down and absorbed into the bloodstream).

Carbohydrates, ATP, and Muscle Contraction

We've established thus far that the first 10 seconds of static contraction exercise require zero in the way of food sources because ATP stores are present in the body and CP stores can create more ATP. After this 10-second point, however, the anaerobic system kicks in with carbohydrates as the primary source of fuel and manufactures its own ATP for the next 50 seconds. After that, the aerobic system begins to kick in.

Our goal with Static Contraction Training is to engage in purely anaerobic activity at the highest possible level of intensity in order to make maximum gains in muscle mass. When the intensity of an exercise is at (or even near) maximal levels during the 10-second anaerobic time frame, the anaerobic system is suddenly forced to break down large amounts of glucose to form large quantities of pyruvic acid. This can only be blown off by engaging the aerobic system, which converts the pyruvic acid into a compound called acetyl co-A, which is then readily dispersed by the system. Since Static Contraction Training attempts to avoid engaging the aerobic system, the bulk of the pyruvic acid is instead chemically transformed into *lactic acid*, or *lactate*. The formation of lactic acid is, essentially, the beginning of the end—at least in terms of the ability of your muscles to continue contracting. Your muscles and the enzymes that comprise and surround them can only withstand a small amount of lactate before the acid starts to shut down the contraction process. Your muscles will begin to burn, and eventually your contraction will cease.

To review: ATP is created through anaerobic and aerobic systems and is required to allow actin and myosin to fulfill their contractile functions. If you exceed your ATP production capacity, the set is over.

FIBER TYPES

Not to complicate matters, but you ought to know that there are several different types of actin and myosin filaments. In fact, the speed with which a muscle can contract is ultimately dependent upon the type of myosin

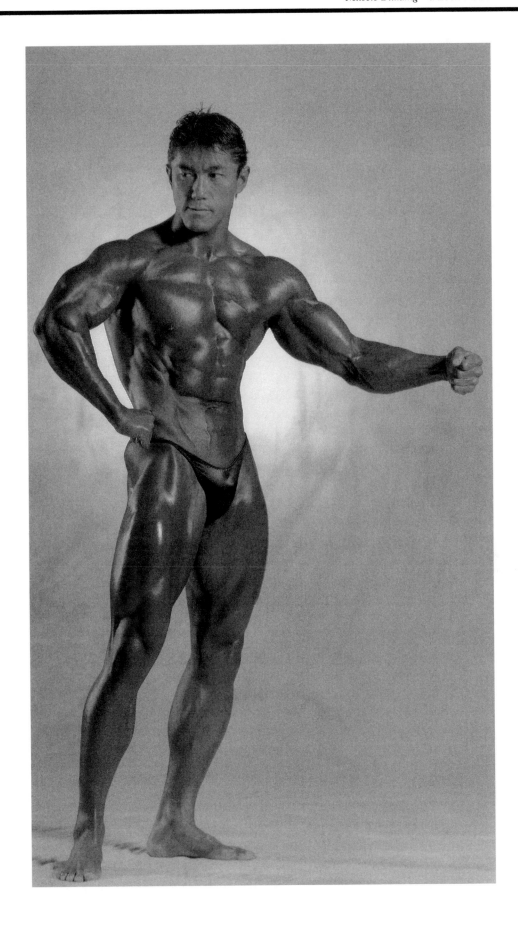

contained within the muscle. Heavy meromyosin (HMM) is recruited for rapid ATP breakdown and is found in powerful, fast muscles. Conversely, light meromyosin (LMM) is a requisite of slower, more endurance-related muscles.

Human anatomy and physiology studies have revealed that four distinct fiber types exist in our species. Talk to most would-be experts or personal trainers and you'll hear a very simplified (and scientifically incorrect) synopsis that there exist only fast-twitch and slow-twitch muscles. Hey, you want some real news? There are presently believed to be three types of fast-twitch muscles!

Fast muscle fibers differ from their slower cousins in many ways, endurance capacity being one of them. In fact, it's in the endurance area rather than in velocity or speed that their differences become most apparent. The fast-oxidative (FO) fibers have relatively good endurance (the term *oxidative* refers solely to the aerobic machinery within the fast-oxidative fiber itself). Fast-glycolytic fibers (FG) which are very fast in contracting, are very powerful but have nothing to offer in the way of endurance (the term *glycolytic* refers to the anaerobic machinery within the fast-glycolytic fiber itself). As an example, the huge deltoids and massive triceps and biceps of Mr. Olympia–caliber bodybuilders are comprised almost entirely of FG fibers.

Intermediate in speed, endurance, and power are the fast-oxidative-glycolytic (FOG) fibers, which contain both the anaerobic and aerobic machinery within their cellular makeup. On the other side of the coin, slow muscle (S), so called because in comparison with, say, FG fibers, they appear thus, is an endurance fiber used primarily by those who engage in distance activities. It's very powerful aerobically with lots of aerobic enzymes, blood vessels, and myoglobin (an oxygen-storing endurance compound). On the downside, however, these fibers aren't capable of creating much force and, consequently, don't possess the inherent mass potential of their quicker cousins.

The Genetic Factor—Again

All right, so what does all of this mean? Well, for those of us with an athletic bent, our fiber type percentages and distribution appear to be genetically predetermined, a product of breeding as opposed to environmental influences, if you will. Still, most of us are brought into the world with a more or less even distribution of all types of fibers, both fast- and slow-twitch. This is not good if you want to be a powerlifter, as obviously a higher complement of FG fibers would be of greater benefit here. But then some of us were born to be marathoners, not sprinters. As a result, premier power-lifters have a high FG fiber percentage, while distance runners have a greater complement of S fibers.

STATIC CONTRACTION AND MUSCLE FIBER RECRUITMENT

Now that we understand how muscles contract, we need to understand the law of muscle fiber recruitment as it pertains to Static Contraction Training. The brain tends to recruit more fibers as it perceives the need for them. This is

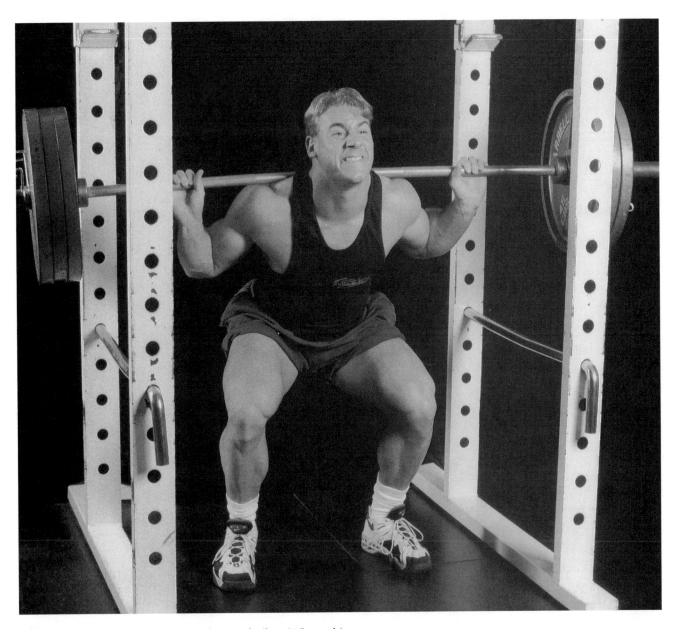

A full-range movement requires using a lighter weight (here 315 pounds).

accomplished via the brain's motor nerves, which, in keeping with the dictates of the brain, follow a relatively fixed order in their recruitment process. The process involves only the precise amount of electrical current necessary to turn on the selected muscle fibers.

Of the four fiber types, the S fibers are the easiest to engage as they don't require a lot of current. Slightly more juice is required to engage the FO fibers and still more for the FOGs. The ones that require the highest electrical output to engage are the FGs. It's important to remember while experiencing the lactic acid slowly building up in the muscle you're training to stick it out for the full 10 seconds. The brain is in no hurry to hit the switch for those FG

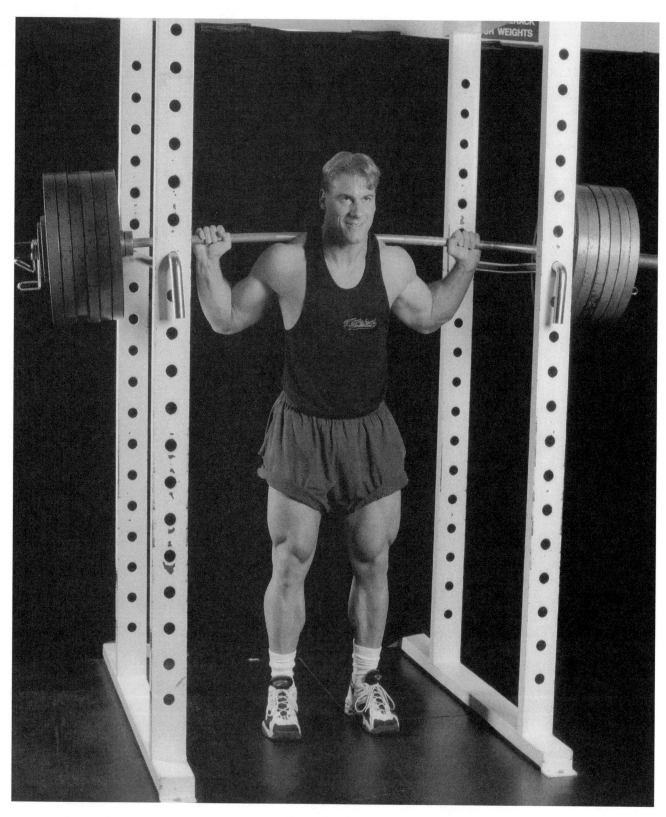

A strong-range movement permits the use of heavier weights that stimulate more muscle fibers (here 600 pounds). That's 600 pounds being lifted by the same muscles! And the scrs proves that the distance the weight is moved is irrelevant to growth stimulation.

fibers—the ones you want to stimulate for size and strength increases. The brain would rather engage the least amount necessary to accomplish a given task, as it is an organ of survival and conserving energy.

The brain will first attempt to accomplish the sustained contraction of a given muscle with only the S fibers. When these soon become inadequate to sustain the contraction, the brain will recruit the FOs and shortly thereafter the FOG fibers to assist with the task. If these fail, and they will, the brain will realize that it needs far more firepower than it's been providing—and only then will it send out the signal to engage the elusive FG fibers. This process is known in physiology circles as *orderly recruitment*, for the brain will not fire up random fibers.

Now it should be clear that the brain, when recruiting muscle fibers, doesn't concern itself with issues of velocity—only force requirements. It has no concern with how quickly you want to lift a weight or to run—remember, it cannot randomly recruit muscle fibers. Instead, the brain ascertains the precise force required to accomplish the task at hand and recruits only the precise amount of muscle fibers accordingly. An important aspect of this phenomenon is that when the brain sends sufficient current to activate the FG fibers during a maximum static contraction, we automatically know that the S, FO, and FOG fibers have been activated and engaged, thereby ensuring maximum muscle fiber stimulation. In other words, if you make your muscles contract against the heaviest weights they are capable of—on a progressive basis—you will have done all that is required to activate all available muscle fibers and stimulate ongoing increases in muscle mass. Any other consideration in this regard is superficial.

REFERENCES

1. Hettinger, T., and E. A. Muller. 1953. "Muskelleistung and Muskel-Training." *Arbeitsphysiologie*. 15:11–126.

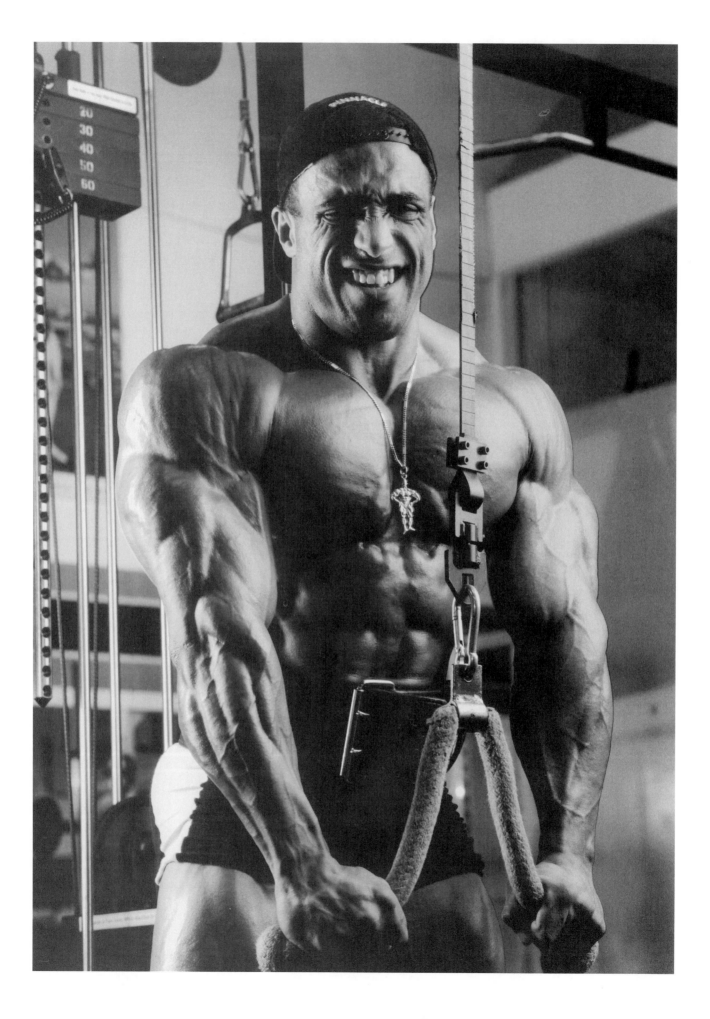

5

Theoretical Principles of Static Contraction Training

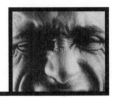

When using Static Contraction Training, you must throw out all preconceived notions of training methodology. You will no longer use repetitions to gauge your progress; from now on you will count seconds. You will no longer look for a variety of exercises to tax the various aspects of a muscle; instead, you will use only one exercise per body part. That one exercise, however, will of necessity employ all of the targeted muscle group's various muscle fibers and stimulate them fully while you contract maximally, until each fiber has been individually and thoroughly spent and you can no longer continue to hold the resistance statically.

THE THEORY

Static Contraction Training is a system that can be grasped by anyone who comprehends the basic tenets behind it. Because most of the material contained herein is based upon empirically validated data, what has worked in the physiology labs can be repeated with equal or greater success by you. We guarantee that if you stick to the program, you will make muscular progress in the space of one month that would have otherwise taken you several years to achieve.

It is essential when embarking upon Static Contraction Training to understand some of the basic physiological principles such as muscle fiber recruitment and the "all or none" principle of muscle fiber contraction in order to reap the full benefits of this training method.

ALL OR NONE

When a muscle contracts, the smallest percentage possible of its available fibers contract maximally and completely, while the rest of the fibers within that muscle do not contract at all. This truth contradicts the common belief that all of a working muscle's fibers contract at once but some to a lesser degree. An individual muscle fiber will contract maximally or not at all.

THE PROBLEM WITH REPETITIONS

In conventional training methods, a typical set sees one arbitrarily choose a given resistance and then bang out as many quick repetitions as possible. As fibers are recruited solely by the amount of weight you are attempting to move, exaggerated arcs or planes of motion with lighter weights limit the amount of stimulation your muscles receive. For example, take a common exercise, the leg extension. You place your legs under the pads of a leg extension machine, lift your legs up until you contract your quadriceps (to full extension), and slowly return to the starting position. Now, at the beginning of the movement you're using only the barest number of muscle fibers. At the halfway point a few more muscle fibers get called into play. Then, at the position of full muscular contraction you've finally done what you set out to do; you're actually forcing a large number of your muscle fibers to get in on the act. However, what typically happens at this point is that long before the fibers can be stressed maximally, the resistance is lowered (often dropped) just as you reach the point of full contraction—and long before the fibers have had time to be fully stressed, giving the momentarily stressed quadriceps muscles a chance to disengage and recover.

Remember that with Static Contraction Training you initiate your set in the position of full muscular contraction—meaning you can use a much heavier weight because you are avoiding the weak range—and keep it there for the duration of your set. It is this methodology that makes this system so effective and separates it from all other training systems.

STATIC CONTRACTION VERSUS ISOMETRICS

Some of you might be thinking, "Oh, I get it—you're contracting your muscles against an immovable object. That's isometrics!" No. This definition does not fit. With Static Contraction Training, your muscles are not pitted against

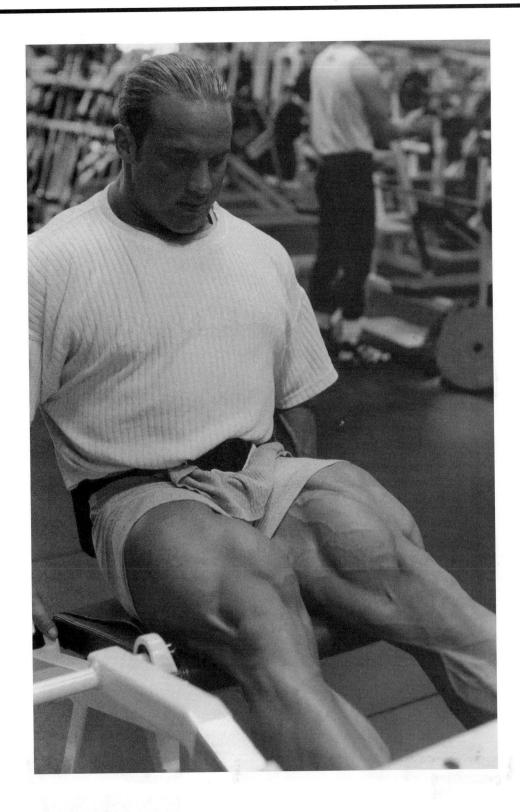

an immovable object, as is the case with isometrics, but rather against a level of resistance that can be measured, quantified, and varied almost infinitely. Plus, the resistance has to be moved into your strongest range before the set can be initiated.

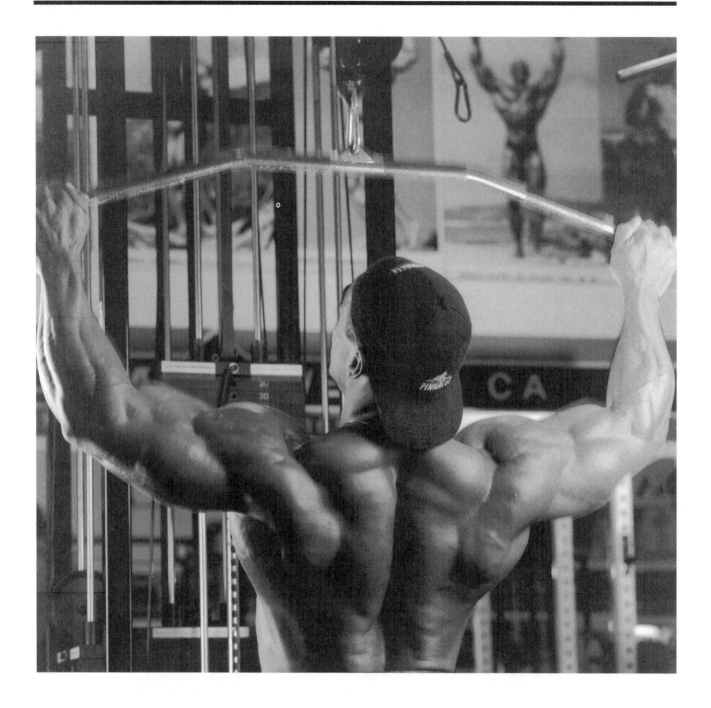

Isometric exercises only initiate contraction in the position where the fewest number of muscle fibers are activated—that is, at the beginning of most movements, such as the bottom quarter of the military press or a "doorknob curl," or the beginning range of a "doorjamb press." The inherent problems with isometric exercises are that they never allow the muscle you're training to progress beyond this minimal level of fiber involvement, and that there is no way of knowing exactly how hard you are pulling on the doorknob or pressing against the doorjamb from workout to workout.

WHY STATIC CONTRACTION IS SO EFFECTIVE

The reason for the dramatic success of Static Contraction Training is simple. Any time movement is involved in exercise, you're simply doing one thing—moving your muscles out of a position of full contraction—which is a step in the wrong direction. Full muscular contraction is the only position in a muscle's range of motion that will accommodate the handling of weights and allow for maximum muscle fiber stimulation to take place. Therefore, anything involving either positive or negative movement, either toward or away from this one strongest-range position involves lower levels of intensity. As has been mentioned, the closer your muscles are to a position of full muscular contraction (wherein a maximal resistance is held statically), the greater the intensity generated and the more muscle fibers you will have activated. The more fibers you stimulate, the more fibers that will grow as a result of having been stimulated. If you're not in a position of full muscular contraction, then you're not involving as many muscle fibers as you could be; and, consequently, you're not stimulating the maximum number of muscle fibers available. As a result, you're not stimulating maximum muscle growth.

In Static Contraction Training all of a given muscle group's fibers are under constant stress or intensity of the highest possible order from the moment the contraction (the "set" in this system) is initiated until its completion 10 to 20 seconds later. This highly efficient technique satisfies the physiological requirements of muscle growth stimulation: maximum fiber involvement and progressive overload without wasted energy in additional low-intensity exercise.

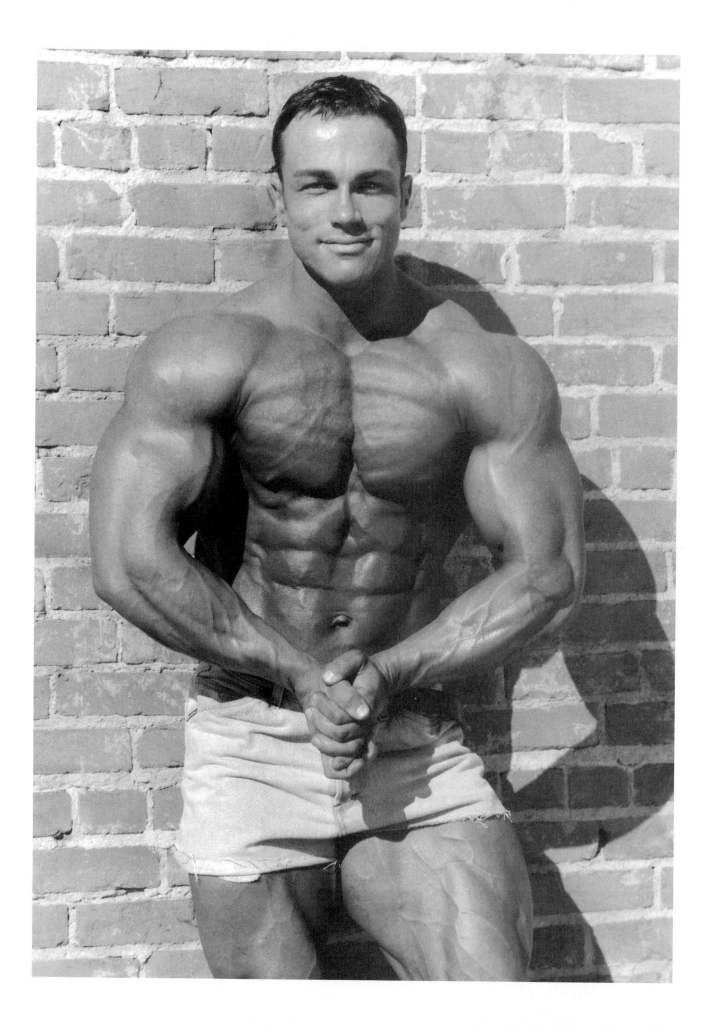

6

The Results of the
Static Contraction Research Study

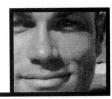

THE SUBJECTS

Volunteer subjects were solicited from our own customer list. Significantly, these were bodybuilders who had been training for up to two years with the Power Factor Training and/or Precision Training systems. That means that they had been training for a long time with ultrahigh intensity and progressive maximal overloads, and had seen some very impressive gains already. Most of them had been training for many years and considered themselves to be near the upper limits of their potential (ranking their muscular development at an average of 6.8 on a scale of 1 to 10). As a group, it would be far more difficult to add new muscle to their bodies than it would for the average person. Further, their average age was 38.4 years! (That's about 20 years older than the test subjects that most training studies use.) We knew that if we could find a way to make these subjects put on new muscle, we'd have a system that would be of enormous value not only to the average person, but even to very experienced bodybuilders.

DOUBLE BLIND

The concept of a so-called "double blind" study is an important and widely used technique in experiments where both the subject's or the test giver's mental attitude could influence the outcome. Double blind techniques are used in drug testing and some psychological tests wherein neither the subject nor the test giver knows any of the objectives of the study or the nature of drugs given. Such a technique cannot be employed in weightlifting. There is no way to get subjects to lift weights without knowing that they are doing it, and there is no way to give them a routine in which they are unaware that they are trying to get stronger or that they are exerting themselves maximally. Our test subjects knew that they were trying to get stronger and we knew we were trying to make them stronger.

CONTROL GROUP

Another technique often used in research studies is to employ a control group. For example, one group of subjects (control group) makes no change whatsoever in its diet, while another otherwise identical group of subjects (test group) changes its protein intake by 300 percent. At the end of the study the two groups are compared for certain characteristics related to protein intake, and observations are made. If we had chosen to have a control group, what strength-training routine would they have performed? Periodization? Heavy-duty? Positions of flexion? Pre-exhaustion? Power Factor Training? See the problem? Instead, we decided that "everybody else" was the control group. For example, regardless of how you normally train, examine the results of the subjects who spent 10 weeks on the SCRS and compare those results to your own progress over the last 10 weeks. In the final analysis, that's all that matters to you anyway: "Will Static Contraction Training work better than what I'm doing right now?"

Static Contraction Research Study (SCRS) Data Summary (Ordered by Lean Mass Gains)

Subject	Average static	Average 1RM	Average 10RM	Transfer of static to full	Sets	Days off between	W/O per week	Lean	Fat	Age	Biceps	Chest	Shoulders	Waist
		Strength (percent gained)				Frequency		Mass (pounds gained)			Size (inches gained)			
Joaquin M.	57.7	16.4	22.1	33.4	3	8.1	0.9	28.9	-18.4	20	0.38	0.75	1.50	0.00
Matt C.	55.9	26.0	47.7	66.0	2	3.1	2.3	21.1	2.9	31	1.00	1.50	0.75	0.00
Gary J.	54.1	34.8	40.6	69.6	2	4.2	1.7	12.7	-10.7	52	0.25	0.00	0.50	-1.00
Kimball M.	36.9	35.0	23.5	79.2	3	2.8	2.5	12.6	-9.6	44	1.00	3.75	0.25	1.25
Shane P.	58.6	25.7	25.9	44.1	3	3.0	2.4	7.8	-0.8	24	0.75	2.00	3.13	1.63
Reg P.	15.7	11.0	12.0	73.4	2	7.1	1.0	6.6	-8.6	50	0.25	0.25	0.50	-2.00
Dave T.	92.4	57.8	69.1	68.7	1	2.6	2.7	6.3	-1.3	44	1.75	3.00	4.00	-2.50
William L.	35.5	12.5	12.2	34.7	3	2.4	2.9	5.6	-9.6	29	0.31	0.63	1.13	-1.00
Michael A.	76.8	60.8	77.1	89.8	2	3.8	1.9	4.1	3.4	34	0.13	-0.50	0.00	0.50
Paul S.	44.2	19.4	19.1	43.5	1	3.7	1.9	2.3	-1.3	51	0.25	0.00	0.00	0.00
Bruce B.	28.1	19.6	20.4	71.1	2	2.3	3.0	1.9	-1.9	44	-0.19	1.50	1.25	-1.25
Tim P.	59.7	12.8	42.3	46.2	2	3.3	2.1	-1.5	-2.5	38	0.50	0.50	1.50	0.00
Averages	51.3	27.6	34.3	60.0	2.2	3.9	2.1	9.0	-4.9	38.4	0.5	1.1	1.2	-0.4

ANALYZING THE DATA

In case the numbers in the table (page 54) do not jump off the page at you, let us state now that these findings are very significant! There were substantial increases in static strength, dynamic full-range strength, lean mass, and muscle size.

Strength Gains

Every one of the subjects in the SCRS had an increase in strength. Their average static strength (measured on 17 different exercises) increased 51.3 percent and, in what will come as a major surprise to virtually everyone, their dynamic strength (over a conventional full range of motion) also increased dramatically.

Aristotle Meets Galileo—Again

As usual, more facts mean fewer myths. Ever heard this one? "When you exercise a muscle statically at only one point, you only get stronger at that limited range. Your static strength gains won't transfer to full-range strength gains." In fact, that's not just a myth, it's the orthodox teaching in every exercise physiology class—anyone with a degree in exercise physiology will tell you that static strength will not transfer to dynamic strength. But 100 percent of the subjects in this study had a positive, significant transference to full-range strength from the gains they made in static strength. The transference averaged 60 percent (see the figures under the heading "Transfer of static to full" in the table on page 54). That means that a person who added 100 pounds to his static bench press would, on average, add 60 pounds to his full-range 1RM and his 10RM!

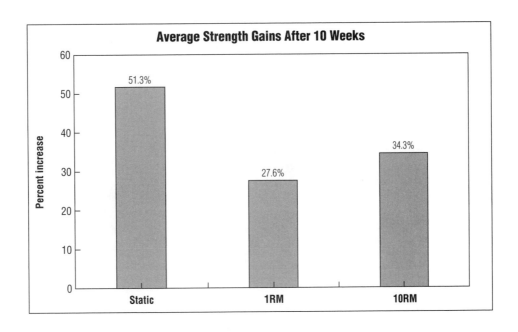

This reminds us of how Aristotle declared that heavier objects fall at a faster acceleration rate than lighter objects. That "law" was taught at the finest universities in the world for nearly 2,000 years. Check the box on the exam that says "same rate" and you flunked. Finally, Galileo decided to actually test this "law" by rolling objects down inclined planes. Sure enough, objects of all weights fell at the same rate of acceleration. Remember that story when you tell an incredulous fellow bodybuilder that training statically will increase your full-range strength. Better yet, be like Galileo and test for yourself.

The Importance of Range of Motion

Here's another bit of institutionalized mythology: "You need a full range of motion in the muscle in order to stimulate growth!" Guess what? Range of motion has an importance somewhere between very little and none. Every gain in mass, strength, and size achieved by everyone in the SCRS was earned with no range of motion whatsoever! Look at Joaquin M.—28.9 pounds of new muscle with *zero* range of motion (see the table on page 54). Think about that, zero range—28.9 pounds of muscle gained. The fact is that substantial gains can be made with no movement (static contraction), some movement (partials by 20,000 Power Factor trainees), and full movement (conventional training). Therefore, the range of motion has no significance.

Size and Mass Gains

The figures in the columns for mass and size speak for themselves. Take a look at the following graphs (pages 56 and 57) and ask yourself, when was the last

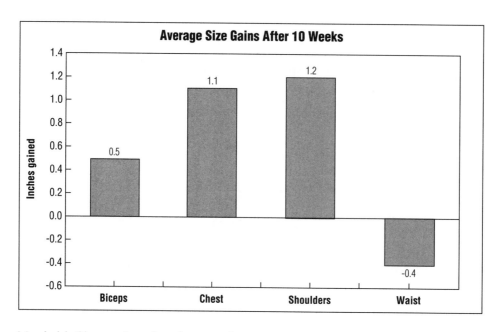

Most bodybuilders spend months in the gym working out and don't see improvement like this. Instead they overtrain week after week.

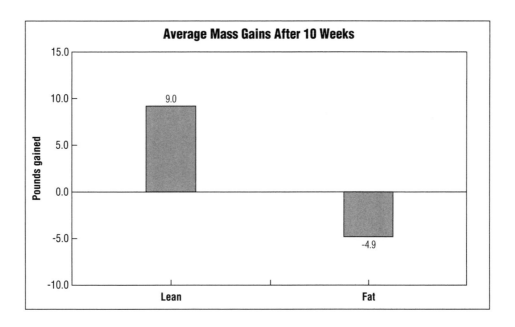

time you had gains like this in 10 weeks of training? Note (in the table on page 54) that only Tim P. had a decrease in muscle mass. We suspect that this is actually the fault of an inaccurate body fat measurement, as his strength increased significantly and his biceps, chest, and shoulders all got bigger—virtually impossible to achieve with a decrease in lean muscle and fat! The likelihood is that Tim P. actually gained muscle and lost even more fat (as his total weight was down four pounds).

Frequency of Training

Much was learned on the subject of training frequency. The table on page 54 shows two columns under the heading "Frequency." These measurements of "Days off between" and "Workouts per week" are actually two ways of expressing the same thing. For example, if you work out one day per week you have seven "Days off between" and one "Workout per week."

Notice that these subjects averaged just 2.1 workouts per week. There was a group that was required to train three days per week. Guess what happened to them? Approximately three weeks into the study, they began to report classic symptoms of overtraining. Some could not continue. Their training schedules had to be altered due to the increasing demands that their strength gains put on their bodies. This proves once again that fixed training schedules like Monday-Wednesday-Friday are useless. If you are getting stronger, you *must* work out less frequently. It's a biological law. Remember Sisco's maxim: "Every day is kidney day." It doesn't make the slightest difference to your kidneys (or liver, or pancreas, or any other internal organ) that yesterday was "leg day" and today is "shoulder day." Growth is systemic, and so is recovery; and although your muscles can get 300 or 400 percent stronger, your kidneys can't. Stronger muscles mean more cleanup work for your kidneys, and since they can't go faster they'll just need more time. Case closed.

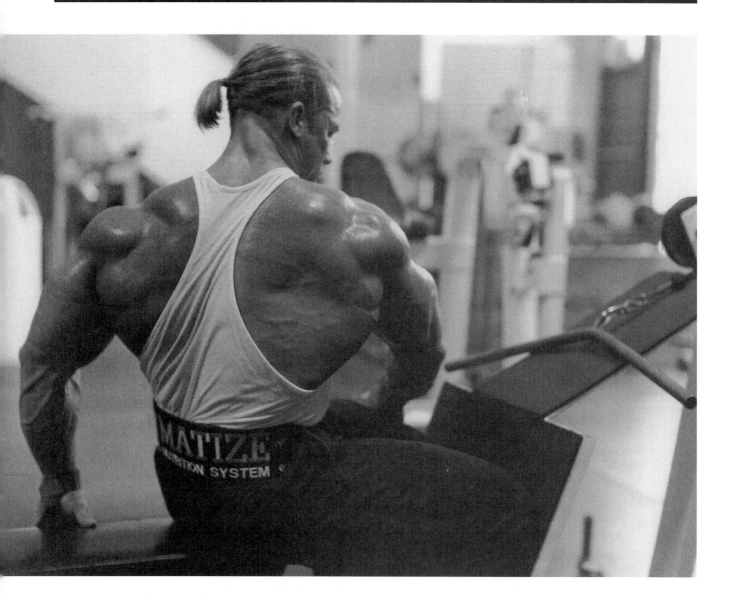

Also, if we compare the top six subjects with the bottom six subjects (ranked by "lean" gains) we see further corroboration of the above trend. The top six subjects worked out, on average, 1.8 times per week. The bottom six worked out 2.4 times per week (33 percent more frequently) but achieved poorer results.

RESULTS OF THE STUDY

The results of this study are very significant. For this group of experienced bodybuilders, averaging age 38.4, to achieve these tremendous increases in mass, strength, and size in only 10 weeks of training is quite possibly without precedent in exercise physiology. That they achieved such results using zero range of motion is certainly unprecedented. Moreover, they have unequivo-

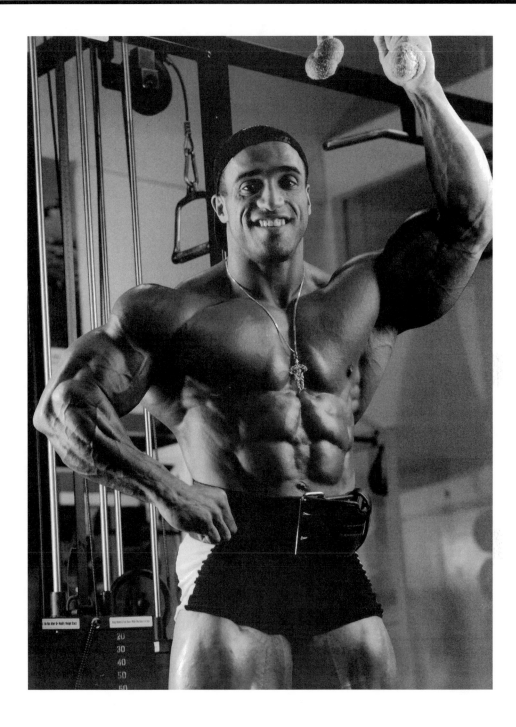

cally proven that, contrary to popular belief, Static Contraction Training does make a very significant contribution to dynamic full-range strength. They have also proved that range of motion has no role in the stimulation of new muscle growth, increased muscle size, or increased strength throughout all ranges of motion.

A quick glance at the average transference number of 60 percent might cause a critic to ask, Why exercise statically if it only yields a 60 percent increase in dynamic transference? There are two answers to this. First, the

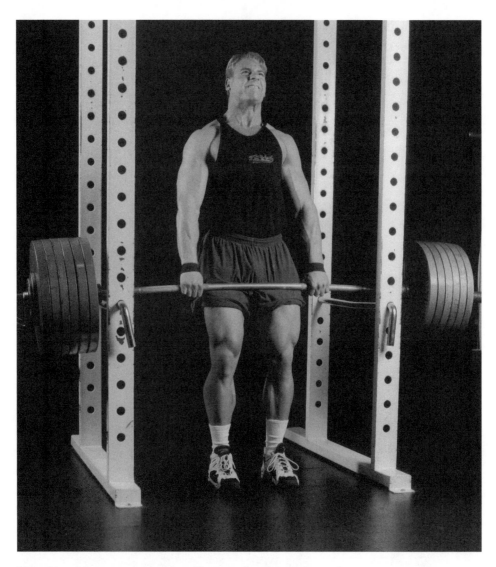

Shrug this weight once a month and you'll never worry about getting weak.

60 percent transference yielded the average subject a 27.6 percent increase in his 1RM and a 34.3 percent increase in his 10RM in 17 different types of lifts. So the question is, Has your conventional training yielded you the same or better increases in dynamic full-range strength over the last 10 weeks? Second, look at the mass and size gains these subjects achieved. Bodybuilders who want more mass and size shouldn't care about which technique they use to get it, even if it means standing on their heads and chanting. Remember, there is nothing sacrosanct about conventional training.

THE SECOND STUDY

Not content with the enormous strides already achieved with the research we've just discussed, we undertook another study involving a different group of subjects. We recruited volunteers from a local golf club. These were people who did not lift weights in any serious manner. We selected four men and four women in their mid-forties to early fifties.

Our purpose was to discover the transference of increased muscle strength to a particular sport skill, in this case the length of a golf drive. (The full results of this study went into our book *The Golfer's Two-Minute Workout*, Contemporary Books.) However, some of the results of this study would be of great interest to bodybuilders and bear repeating here.

Reduced Hold Times

The first study involved hold times of 15 to 30 seconds. As soon as we proved that that was enough time to generate huge muscle mass increases, we wondered if less time would also work. The golfers used hold times of only 10 to 20 seconds. This, as you shall see, was also enough to stimulate huge increases in strength.

Reduced Sets and Frequency

The golfers were put on a program that involved only one set per exercise and averaged only 6.6 workouts over a six-week period. All in all, that's about half of the muscular work performed by the members of the first study.

Results of the Second Study

The second group had huge increases in strength in every exercise. The overall average in all exercises in all test subjects was 84 percent! This, not surprisingly, transferred to enormous improvements in their golf games.

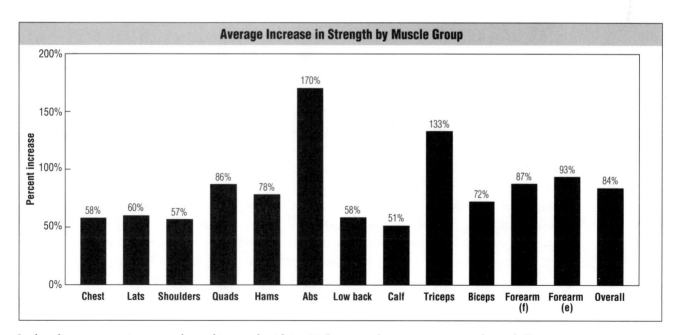

Look at the enormous improvement these subjects made with just 14.5 minutes of exercise over a six-week period. Has your strength gone up this much in the last six weeks?

Percent Increase in Strength Per Muscle Group

	W/O	Total time (min.)	Chest	Lats	Shoulders	Quads	Hams	Abs	Low back	Calf	Triceps	Biceps	Forearm (flexors)	Forearm (extensors)	Overall
Mike M., Sr.	7	14.8	48	47	52	57	129	57	41	52	70	50	38	80	60
Mike M., Jr.	8	17.8	48	129	52	129	64	71	62	106	200	100	57	80	91
Paul R.	9	23.4	63	47	64	100	104	233	45	42	100	67	43	100	84
Steve H.	8	17.2	55	43	27	90	67	100	50	35	75	30	33	67	56
Bonnie H.	5	10.5	70	33	75	73	43	300	50	33	150	50	100	75	88
Joyce L.	4	8.0	33	50	43	62	36	100	55	50	200	63	117	67	73
Kathy M.	6	11.9	93	78	87	91	100	200	80	33	140	133	133	150	110
Laura G.	6	12.1	50	57	53	89	83	300	86	62	125	83	175	125	107
Average	6.6	14.5	58	60	57	86	78	170	58	51	133	72	87	93	84

Average time per workout: 2.2 min.

Training Time of Static Contraction Training Versus Conventional Training

	Bench press	Lat pulldown	Shoulder press	Leg extension	Leg curl	Weighted crunch	Total time (min)
Static contraction workout (15 sec average per exercise)	0.25	0.25	0.25	0.25	0.25	0.25	1.5
Conventional training (3 sets of 12 reps + 1 min between sets)	6.5	6.5	6.5	6.5	6.5	6.5	39.0

Static contraction workout (1 workout per week) 1.5 min
Conventional training (3 workouts per week) 117.0 min

It's difficult to believe that 1 percent of the exercise time of conventional training would yield these results . . . but it is exactly what happened.

The reduced frequency of training improved (!) their gains over the first test group (although the first group was already very well developed). As it happened, the four women in the study averaged only 5.25 workouts in six weeks, compared to the men, who averaged 8 workouts. Yet the women saw a 95 percent increase in overall strength, compared to the men's 73 percent increase. Compare this with the frequency of a conventional Monday-Wednesday-Friday routine that would have imposed 18 workouts over the same six-week period . . . and probably would have generated nearly zero increase in strength.

Look at the graph (page 63) that shows the difference in training time between Static Contraction Training and a very abbreviated conventional routine. The fact is that all subjects using Static Contraction Training saw huge increases in strength and (where measured) muscle mass, yet they were on a program that imposed about 1 percent of the exercise time demands of a conventional workout. Think about that the next time a guy tells you he trains for two hours a day, six days a week. Ask him if his results are 100 to 400 times better than what they would be with Static Contraction Training. Heck, ask him if they're even as good!

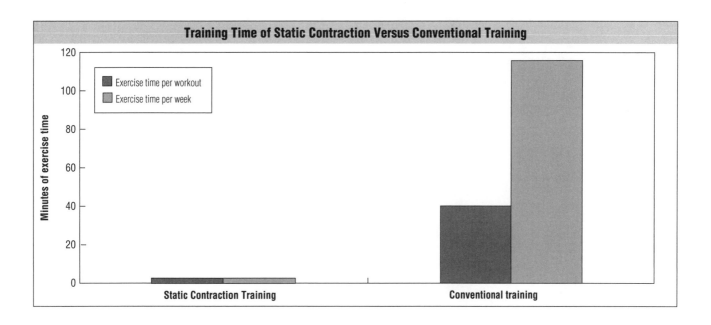

STATIC STRENGTH—WHO NEEDS IT?

It's strange how getting involved in a certain subject has a way of leading to other issues. Our initial interest in Static Contraction Training was its application as a "minimum dose" form of exercise. Not being hard-core bodybuilders or ones who like to spend as much time in the gym as possible or who get a "high" just in anticipation of a workout, we were looking for ways to get more benefit from fewer workouts. For both of us, lifting weights is a means to get stronger; we can then use that strength doing something we enjoy outside of the gym.

Thus, Static Contraction Training's appeal was the fact that it permitted brief workouts that could be spaced far apart. As we are now looking at the taillights of forty, we are particularly interested in the minimum dose of exercise that can trigger new muscle growth *and* sustain lean mass into middle age and beyond.

Old habits of thinking are often difficult to break. Even when we designed the Static Contraction Research Study, we took measurements that would demonstrate static training's benefits not only to static strength and muscle mass gains but also to full-range strength. It's taken some time to realize that static strength has its own merits, which, in many applications, rank above those of full-range strength.

We have become sensitive to how often we find ourselves using the static strength of muscles rather than their dynamic strength. For example, when riding a motorcycle, particularly in off-road conditions, the body expends a great deal of muscular energy mostly through holding the muscles statically. The biceps and triceps hold the handlebars in a more or less fixed position despite being bumped and buffeted by various obstacles. The quadriceps and hamstrings hold the body in a position three or four inches off the seat and

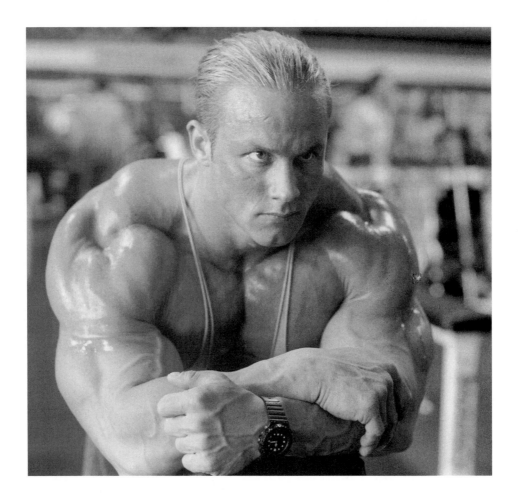

do their best to maintain that rigid position in space despite the up and down motion of the motorcycle.

The value of static strength also becomes apparent while trapshooting. All shooting sports rely on the ability of the muscles to have sufficient static strength to hold the gun perfectly steady under all conditions. Dynamic, or full-range strength, is never used. Pete's 12-year-old son, Alex, can always break more clay pigeons on his first 10 shots than he can on his second 10. This difference can be attributed to the muscle fatigue that sets in some time after those first 10 shots. (The same holds true for most adults after 30 to 50 shots.) There is no doubt that as his static strength increases, he will find it less tiring to hold his shotgun, and his scores will improve proportionately.

Two more examples are water skiing and alpine skiing. A water skier holds his arms and legs in a more or less rigid position while skiing. He will shift position from time to time, but once shifted, his knees and elbows stay bent at about the same angle. Bobbing up and down in the range of motion of a squat, for example, would serve no purpose except to look ridiculous and manifest bad form. Skiers need static strength and they need it at a particular point in their range of motion.

The list of sports and activities that utilize static strength (either fully or partially) is really quite extensive. Horseback riding, mountain biking, wrestling, jet skiing, nearly all types of gymnastics, fencing, and many other sports lend themselves to Static Contraction Training. When an athlete needs more static strength at a specific point in his range of motion, he should exercise statically in order to develop the exact form of strength he needs, where he needs it. And this is what Static Contraction Training does. Not only does it maintain and/or increase muscle mass; it also places additional strength exactly where it is needed and in the form that it is needed.

MORE RESEARCH

We have already begun more experimentation on the limits of reducing exercise time and frequency. We have personally engaged in an eight-week study involving only five workouts. As this study unfolds and rest periods are constantly increased, it will require only seven workouts in the course of an entire year, provided that we show some amount of improvement in every workout. Already, in only five workouts we have seen our weights increase in the shrug exercise from 360 and 450, respectively, to 750 and 1,000. High rows on a Hammer Strength machine have gone from 450 and 540, respectively, to 830 and 900 pounds. And this has been done with hold times of just 5 seconds! This means that 25 seconds of muscle stimulation on each exercise spread over an eight-week period has led to just over a 100 percent increase in strength . . . and we weren't exactly weak little kittens when we started.

In summary then, we have established that neither full-range exercise nor frequent trips to the gym are necessary in an efficient strength- and size-building program. In fact, tremendous gains can be obtained with workouts lasting as briefly as 20 seconds (total training time) and performed only once every two weeks.

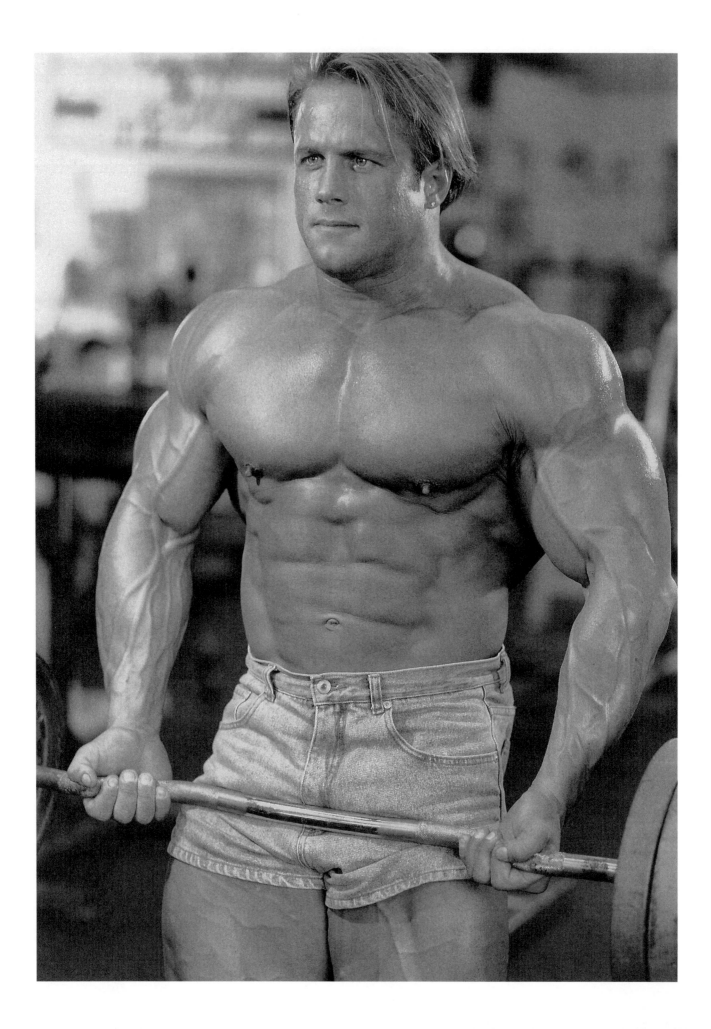

7

The Static Contraction Workout

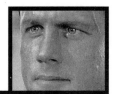

This chapter contains our recommendation of the most efficient, effective static contraction workout. Please keep in mind that whenever we work with averages we are engaging in a measure of compromise. There is tremendous variation among individuals; so, as always, the watchwords are *maximum intensity* and *progressive overload*. Above all, keep those objectives in mind.

STATIC CONTRACTION DEFINED

What is a static contraction? Your muscles are statically contracted when they are holding a weight in a "locked" position but remaining motionless. For example, if a person stands at attention, his knees are locked so that his weight is carried by his bones. He can stand like that all day with little muscular fatigue. However, if he bends his knees, his leg muscles take over the task of holding him motionless. His muscles are under severe load stress, but they are not moving up and down. This is a static contraction, and it is a very demanding form of overload.

RANGE OF MOTION

In every exercise, there is a range through which you could choose to move the weight. For example, in the bench press you could hold the weight one inch off your chest, or one inch from lockout, or anywhere in between (in other words, anywhere from your weakest range to your strongest range). In Static Contraction Training, all of the exercises should be performed in your strongest range—but *do not* fully lock out during the exercise time period.

TIMEKEEPING AND REPS

As you should know by now, time is a critical element in the measurement of strength and of exercise intensity. Fortunately, this static contraction routine will be the simplest routine that you have ever trained with in this regard. Since there are no reps, your entire set consists of holding the weight motionless for 5 to 15 seconds. This time period was chosen as a middle ground from all of our research so far.

Progress is made by using the same weight until you can hold it for 15 seconds. Once a 15-second static contraction has been achieved, increase the weight by 15 to 30 percent to find the weight that you can statically hold for 5 seconds. Every "set" will consist of holding the weight for a duration between 5 and 15 seconds.

For example, suppose that you can bench press (in a static contraction) 100 pounds for 5 seconds. You would remain with 100 pounds in your next workout but try to hold it for 9 seconds, or 13 seconds, or whatever increase you can achieve. When you are able to hold 100 pounds for a full 15 seconds, it is time to increase the weight. The percentage of increase will vary among individuals, so you will have to experiment a bit to determine how much of an increase you can handle. Suppose you can now hold 125 pounds for 5 seconds. You would continue to use 125 pounds until you can hold it for 15 seconds, then start all over with a higher weight for 5 seconds.

Since you are holding all sets to failure, you will occasionally have a time that is slightly outside the workout parameters, such as 3 seconds or 22 seconds. That's OK as long as it only happens occasionally—some variation is normal and expected (and it shows that you are really testing your limits).

SETS

You will be performing only one set per exercise. It is likely that a minority of individuals would see slightly better results (10 percent or so) by performing a second set. However, this is 100 percent more work for a very small increase in progress that might not even happen. Time and again we are learning that less is more in strength training. Go for an all-out, maximum-intensity set without having to think about saving energy for a second set.

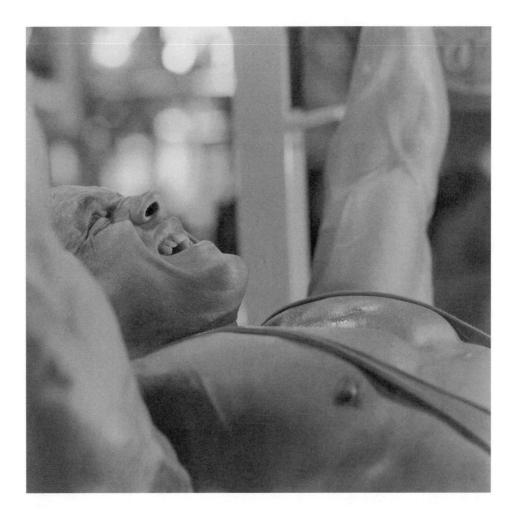

WRITE IT DOWN

You will make much better progress over the long term if you have a log that contains the specifics of each workout. (See page 17, Chapter 3, for more on these logs.) Progressive overload is an indispensable condition of making gains—and unless you have a photographic memory, you won't remember how many seconds you held your squat four weeks ago. It is really a very simple task to write down the weight and number of seconds for only five exercises.

IMPORTANT SAFETY NOTE

It is critically important to limit the range of motion of the weight you are using. If you do not have a strong partner who can spot you during your lifts and who is capable of lifting any weight you are using, then you *must* use a power rack, Smith machine, or other device to prevent the weight from moving into your weak range. Lifting heavy weight is perfectly safe under these conditions, provided you keep the weight under control. In fact, Static

Contraction Training involves an extra margin of safety because it involves no motion of the weight.

EXERCISE DESCRIPTIONS

Workout A

Standing Barbell Press (Shoulder Press)
This movement can be performed either seated or standing. If performed seated with a universal machine, place a stool between the handles of the

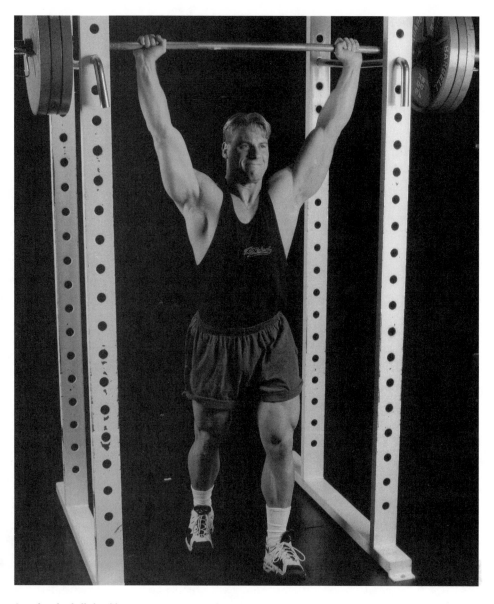

Standing barbell shoulder press in a power rack.

shoulder press station of the machine. Sit on the stool facing toward the weight stack, locking your legs around the uprights of the stool to secure your body in position. If performed standing while utilizing a universal machine, assume a split stance. Taking an overgrip on the handles attached to the lever arm of the station, have a partner assist you in lifting the handles upward to straight arms' length overhead. Lower the handlebars slightly, and hold this position for 5 to 15 seconds.

If performing this exercise with free weights, do so in a power rack or Smith machine. Adjust the height of your support so that the bar is about two inches below the height of a fully extended rep. From a standing position, with your hands approximately three inches wider on each side than your shoulders, press the bar upward until your elbows are locked. Lower the bar slightly, just enough to break the lock in your elbows, and hold for 5 to 15 seconds.

Cable Row for Lower Back

Sit in the rowing position in front of the low pulley. Lean forward and grasp the handles of the low cable. Keeping your elbows straight (but not locked), use the muscles of your lower back to recline to an angle of approximately 45 degrees. Be sure to avoid using the muscles of your arms to pull the weight. Hold this position for 5 to 15 seconds.

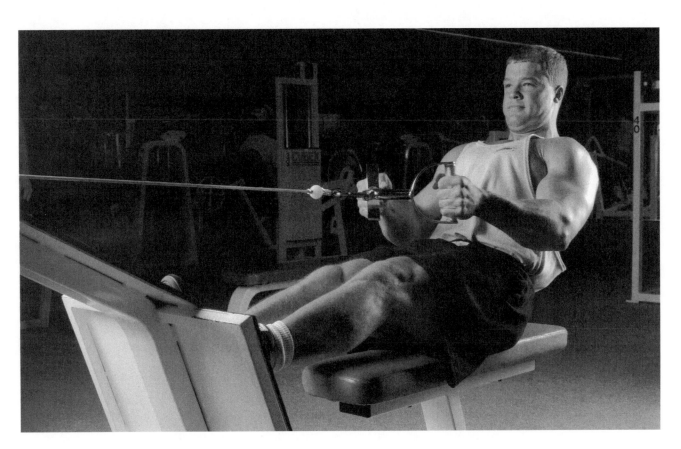

Cable row for lower back.

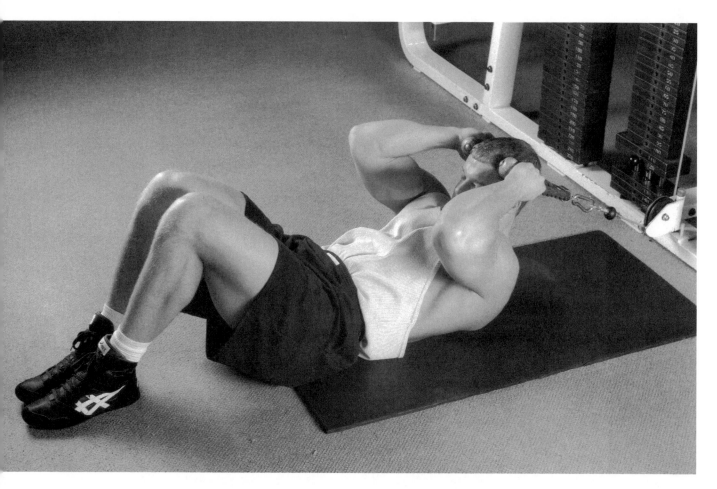

Weighted crunch—the single best ab exercise we've ever found! (That's 120 pounds he's crunching!)

Weighted Crunch

To begin, lie on your back on the floor, hands behind your head, and feet flat on the floor or anchored beneath a secure object. Take hold of the crunch strap or the curling handle of a low pulley unit and, while trying to keep your chin on your chest, slowly curl your trunk upward toward a sitting position. Make sure you hold onto the strap tightly so that your abdominals are contracting maximally against the resistance. You'll find that you can only curl up one-third of the range you would if performing a conventional sit-up. This is fine because that is all the range of motion that your abdominals require to be stimulated to grow stronger. Once you have ascended to a fully contracted position, hold this position for 5 to 15 seconds.

Bench Press

Start by lying on your back on a flat bench. If utilizing a universal machine bench press, have your partner assist you in lifting the handlebars upward until your arms are fully extended. From this position, bend your elbows slightly so that the resistance is lowered one to two inches. Hold this position for 5 to 15 seconds.

If you are using free weights, make sure that you do all of your lifting inside a power rack. Set the pins in the rack to three to four inches below your full lockout reach. Place your feet flat on the floor for balance. Your grip should be medium width, so that as you lower the bar your forearms are straight up and down (vertical). Raise the barbell from the pins and lock it out directly above your chest. With the bar directly above your chest, lower the bar until there's a slight bend in your elbows—not such a bend that the barbell touches the pins in the power rack, but enough that it comes close to touching—and hold this position for 5 to 15 seconds.

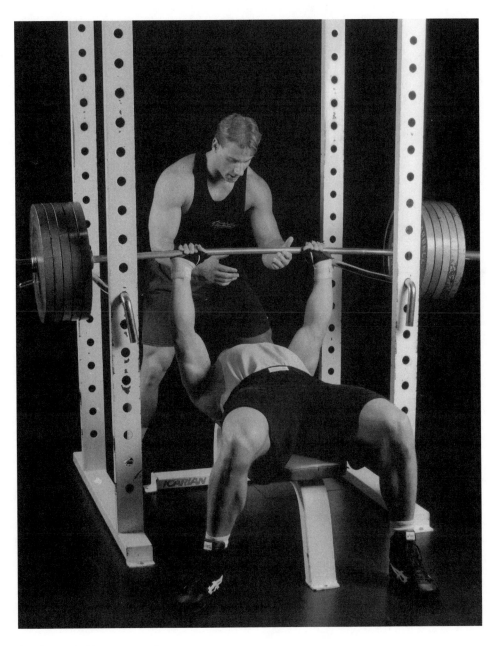

Bench press inside a power rack.

Barbell Shrug

Stand inside a power rack or Smith machine and adjust the bar so it is only one to three inches below your reach. Grasp the bar with an overhand grip that is approximately shoulder width. Raise the bar off the supports, then shrug your shoulders up and hold this position for 5 to 15 seconds.

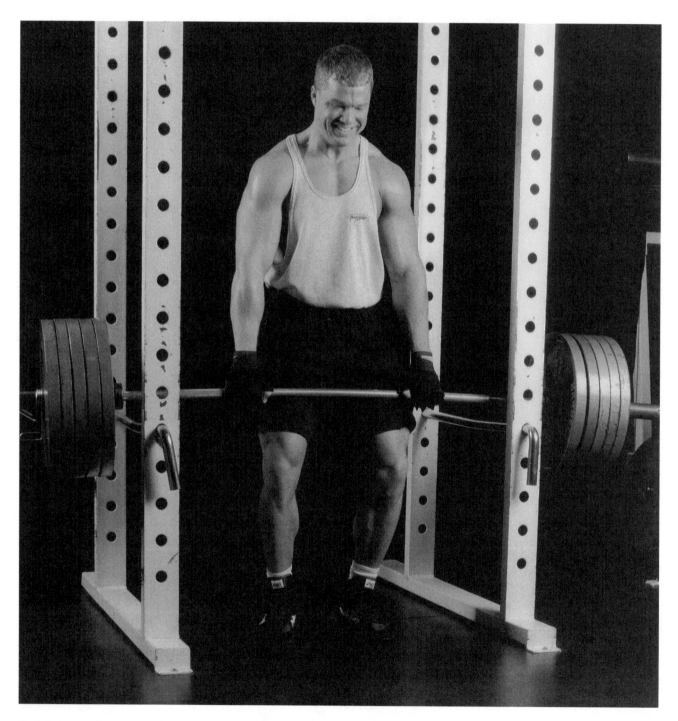

Barbell shrug inside a power rack.

Workout B

Lat Pulldown

To begin, take a close underhand grip on the bar. Sit either on the floor or on a seat with your knees hooked under the support. Your arms should be stretched fully above your head, and you should feel the pull mostly in your lats and somewhat in your biceps. Pull the bar just slightly down—about two to three inches—and hold this position for 5 to 15 seconds. (Note: When your strength exceeds the limit of the weight stack, this movement can be performed unilaterally by attaching a pulley handle to the lat bar attachment and pulling down with one arm for 5 to 15 seconds, and then repeating the procedure with the opposite arm.)

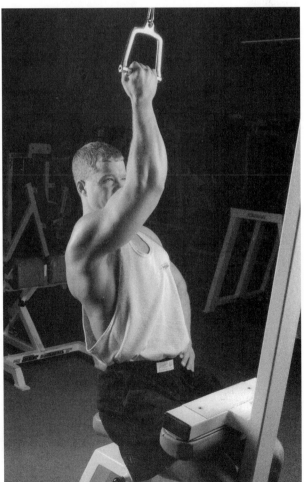

Lat pulldown.

One-armed lat pulldown.

Close-Grip Bench Press
This is performed in the same manner as the bench press, except that your hands should be spaced only four inches or so apart. This places the emphasis of the exercise directly on the triceps.

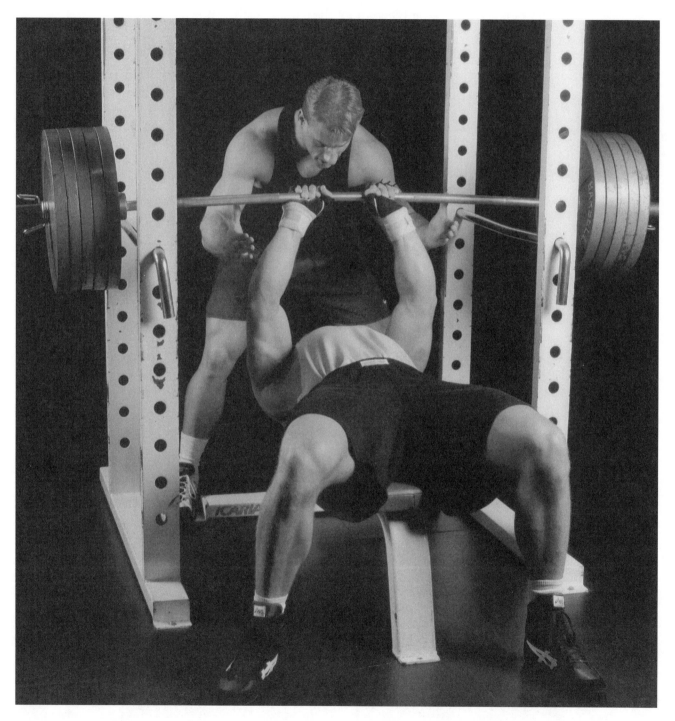

Close-grip bench press inside a power rack. Notice how the weight cannot descend more than about three inches? It is virtually impossible to get injured with this form of training.

Cable Curl

Stand in front of the low pulley with your feet spaced shoulder-width apart. Take an underhand grip on the curl bar. Position your body so that your arms are bent at about 90 degrees when you start the movement. Pull back on the bar to raise the weight stack two inches. Hold this position for 5 to 15 seconds.

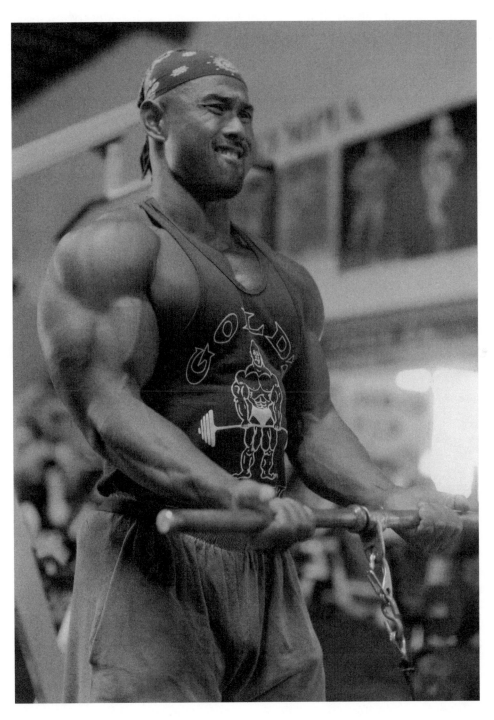

Cable curl.

Leg Press

Sitting down on the padded seat, brace your back against the upper back pad and adjust the seat position so that your legs, when placed upon the foot pedals, are only slightly bent (nearly fully extended). Leaving the safety stops in place so the weight won't descend, place your feet flat on the platform and slowly press forward until your legs are one inch from being fully extended. Hold it for 5 to 15 seconds. (Note: This movement can be performed unilaterally as well, by simply lifting the resistance with both legs and then removing one leg from the platform. Hold for 5 to 15 seconds per leg.)

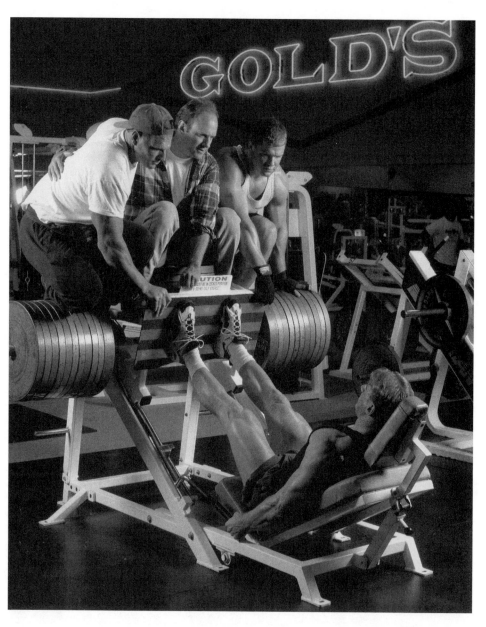

Leg press. OK, don't do this at your gym—but this 2,000+ pound lift is what many people are capable of lifting when using Static Contraction Training.

Toe Press

Sitting down on the padded seat, brace your back against the upper back pad and adjust the seat position so that your legs, when placed upon the foot pedals, are only slightly bent (nearly fully extended). Leaving the safety stops in place so the weight won't descend, place the balls of your feet firmly on the footrests and slowly press forward until your calves are in a fully contracted position. Hold it for 5 to 15 seconds. (Note: This movement can be performed unilaterally as well by simply lifting the resistance with both legs and then removing one leg from the foot pedal so that the calf muscle of the remaining leg is bearing the full resistance. Hold for 5 to 15 seconds per leg.)

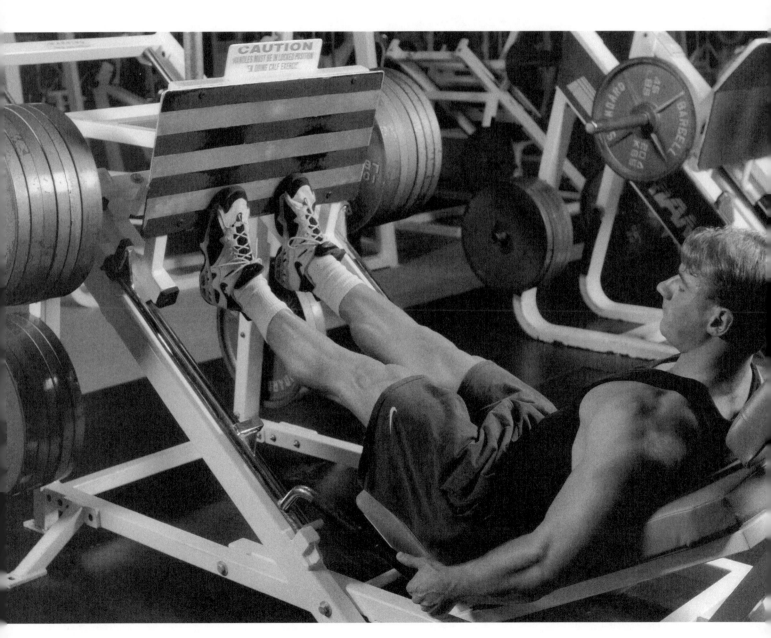

Toe press.

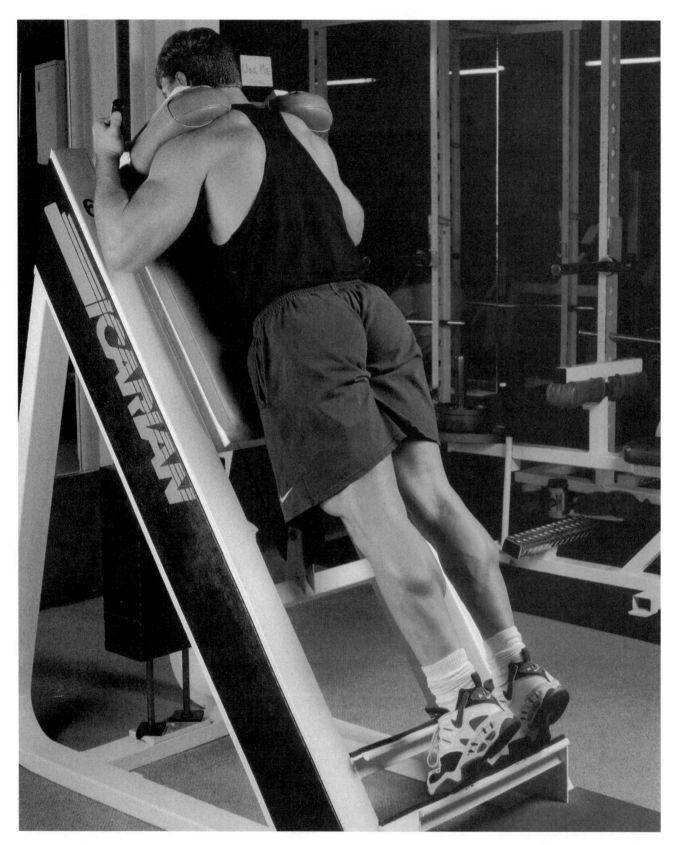

Toe press on Hack squat machine.

ALTERNATE EXERCISES

Virtually any exercise can be utilized in a static contraction manner. While the above exercises make up the short list of the best exercises for producing high overload and great results, there are many other exercises that we have found productive. All of the following exercises have been used with success in Static Contraction Training:

- Nautilus lower back machine or barbell deadlift instead of cable row for low back
- Cable pressdown or weighted dip instead of close-grip bench press for triceps
- Preacher curl or machine curl instead of cable curl for biceps

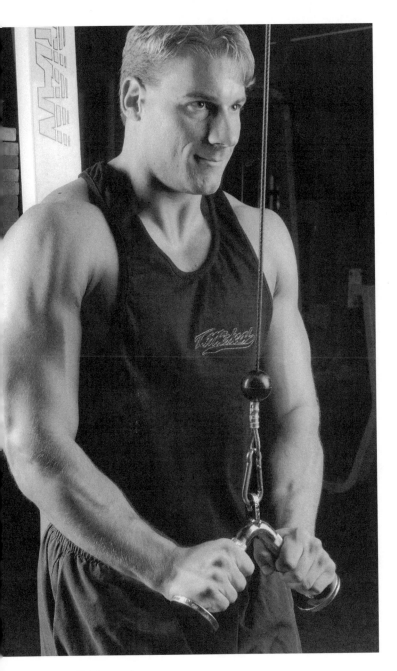

Cable pressdown.

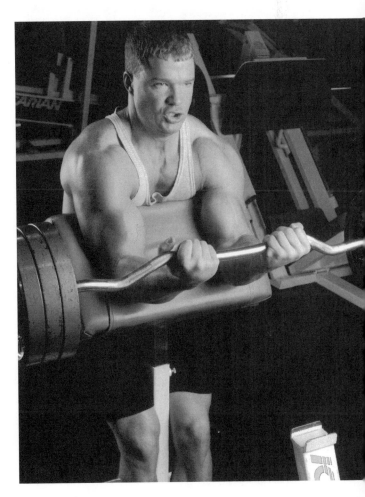

Preacher curl.

- Wrist curl and reverse wrist curl—good for tennis players, golfers, and other athletes who want an extra measure of forearm power
- Squats, leg extension, and leg curl—all excellent choices in static contraction leg training

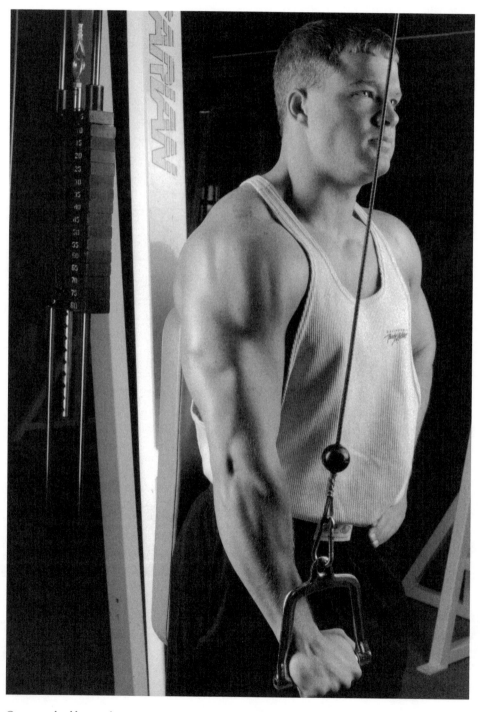

One-armed cable pressdown.

- Seated row using no back movement and only the lats to raise the weight two inches—a great alternative to lat pulldowns

If you decide to do some experimentation, remember to always choose the exercise that permits you to use the most weight for a particular muscle. For example, if you can perform a 10-second hold with 120 pounds in the cable pressdown but 200 pounds for 10 seconds in a close-grip bench press, stick with the close-grip bench press as it will stimulate more growth.

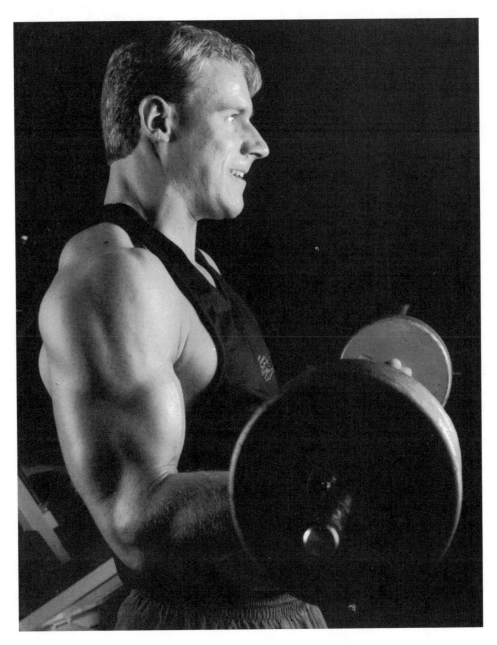

Standing barbell curl.

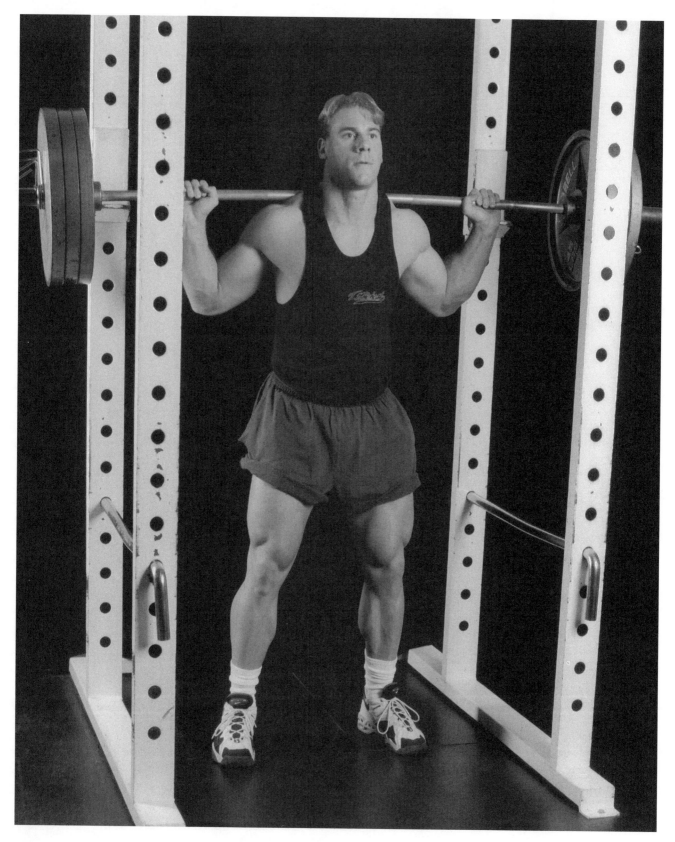

Barbell squat.

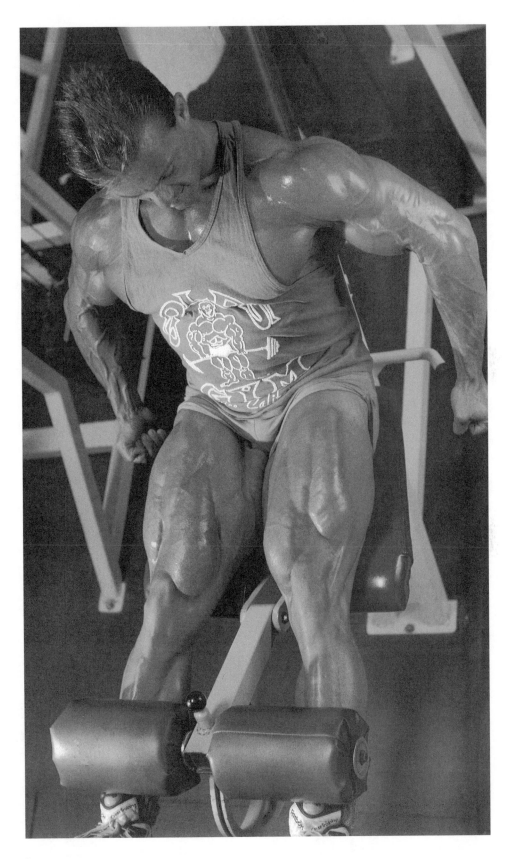

Leg extension.

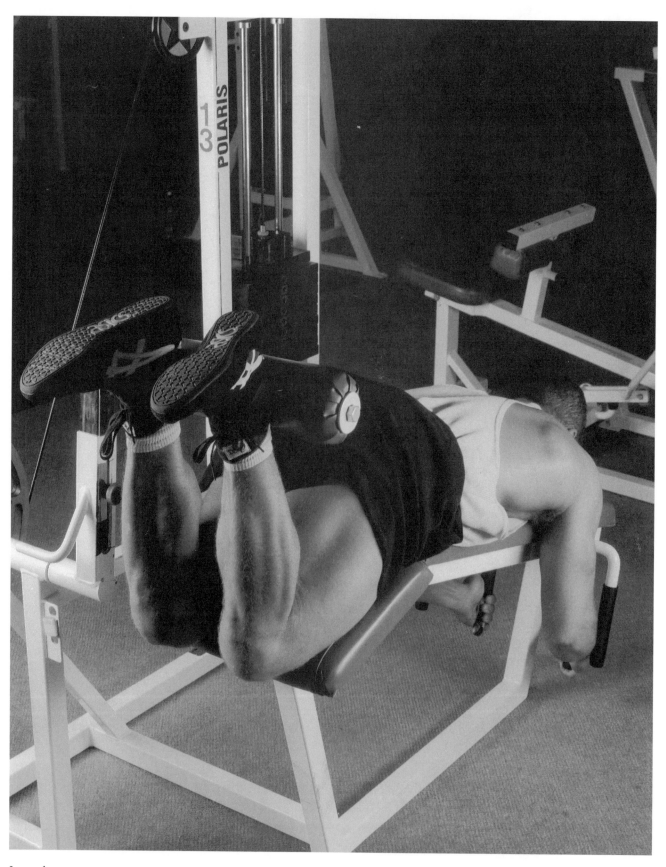

Leg curl.

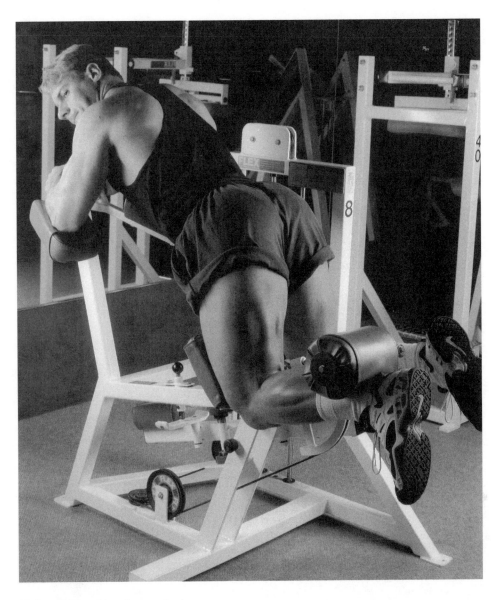

Unilateral leg curl (one leg at a time).

POINTS TO KEEP IN MIND

- Train with a partner, or use a power rack or Smith machine to limit the movement of the weight.
- Hold the weight between 5 and 15 seconds only.
- Use weights that are heavy enough to cause total muscular fatigue within the 5 to 15 seconds.
- Perform each exercise only once per workout.
- Space workouts far enough apart to ensure progress in every workout.
- Count only static time—do not keep the clock running while the weight descends.

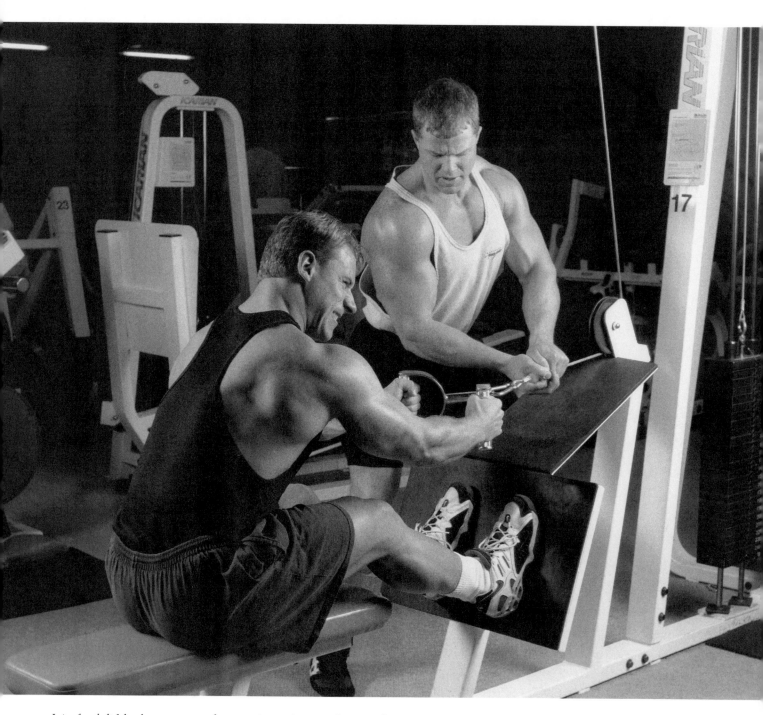

It is often helpful to have a partner who can assist you in moving heavy weights into your strongest range.

FREQUENCY OF TRAINING

Alternate the two workouts—for example, Monday A, Thursday B, Monday A, Thursday B, and so on. If you are a total beginner to weight training, you can begin this program on a two-day-per-week schedule (for example, Monday and Thursday or Tuesday and Friday), but you can only stay on it for two or three weeks. After three weeks, switch to a one-per-week schedule. (For example, Monday the 1st A, Monday the 8th B, Monday the 15th A, and so on.) If you are not a total beginner, you should begin by training only once per week. However, in every case, you should pay attention to your progress and be willing to adjust your training frequency. (This is the single most important factor in your long-term progress!)

To know how and when to adjust your individual workouts and your training frequency, just follow these two simple rules:

1. If, on any workout, you fail to make progress on three out of five exercises, it's time to add an extra three days off between all workouts from now on. Don't just add three days off "this time." Your body has grown to a new level of power, and your workouts will be so demanding that you will need more time off after every workout.

2. If, on any workout, you fail to make progress on one or two exercises, you need to skip those exercises next time you perform the same workout. Just do the three or four remaining exercises next time you do the same workout. When you add them back in, you will find your strength has increased during the extended rest for those muscle groups.

Follow these two rules to the letter, and you will experience growth like you never have before. The worst thing you can do is decide for yourself that these few seconds of total muscular overload will not be enough and start adding other routines and programs into your training. This system has already been tested on hundreds of athletes and bodybuilders, and we know it works in 100 percent of cases. Never forget that intensity versus duration graph (see page 21). This program is designed to deliver maximum intensity and minimum duration—let it do just that.

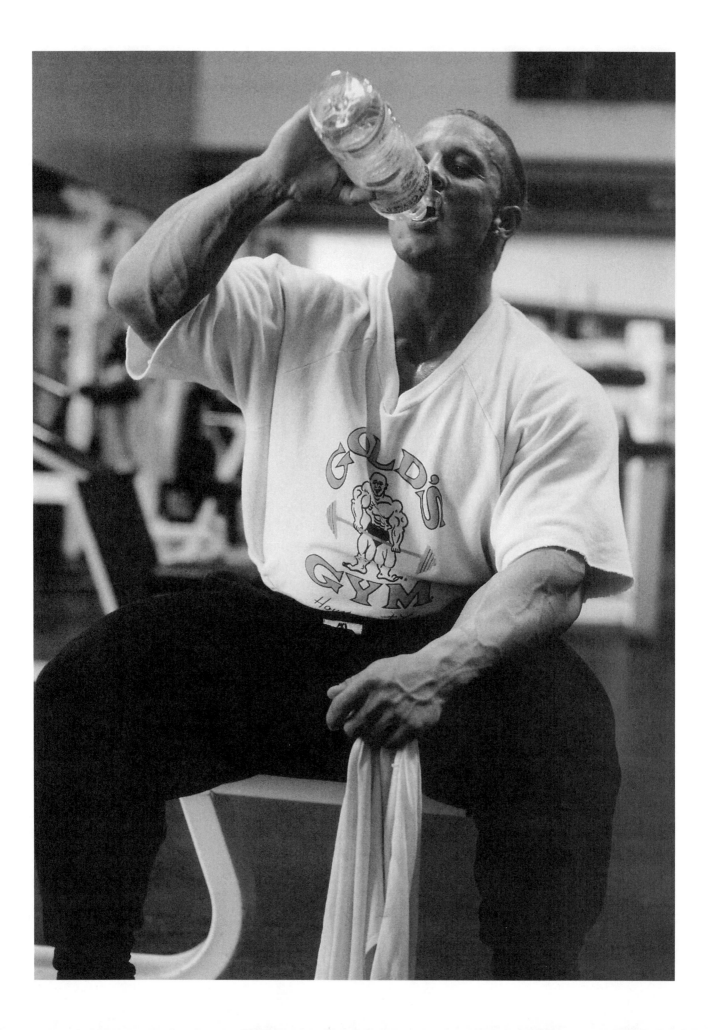

8

Optimal Nutrition for Static Contraction Training

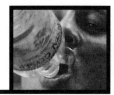

Static Contraction Training places unusual stresses on the body's various biochemical reserves. These reserves include the amino acid pool (which is of vital significance since amino acids are the very stuff of life and of big muscles); the elements sodium and potassium, electrolytes needed for high-intensity muscle contraction; those important minerals, calcium and magnesium, which help maintain a steady-state nervous system; and vitamins, which transform our food into the enzymes responsible for energy metabolism. These nutrients are but a few that go into making up a well-balanced diet. Without an ample supply each day of protein, vitamins, minerals, fats, carbohydrates, and water, your workouts will inevitably degenerate into pointless affairs, full of sound and fury perhaps, but ultimately signifying nothing.

THE VARIOUS NUTRIENTS

The first requisite for building a championship physique is health. Along with adequate rest, maintaining a well-balanced diet is absolutely essential in developing your physique. Balancing your diet for health maintenance and for muscle gains requires over 40 different nutrients. These various nutrients can be obtained from generous daily portions of the four basic food groups:

- Cereals and grains
- Fruits and vegetables
- Milk and dairy products
- Meat, fish, and poultry

The various nutrients are classified within the six major categories already mentioned: protein, vitamins, minerals, fats, carbohydrates, and water. The following analysis will help you understand the role of each in your muscle building diet:

Protein: The word *protein* is derived from the Greek word *protos*, meaning first. The primary constituent of muscle tissue (after water), protein makes up the bulk of the contractile element within muscle.

Carbohydrates: The primary fuel source of our muscles comes from carbohydrates in the simple form known as glucose. When we don't take in enough sugar through our diets to fuel muscular contractions, our bodies transform the amino acid alanine, derived from ingested protein of our own muscle tissue, into glucose. So carbohydrates have a protein-sparing effect. In addition to supplying energy, carbohydrates supply important building blocks of life as well. Deoxyribose, found in RNA and DNA (two essential components of all living matter), is a form of sugar derived from the carbohydrates we eat. Carbohydrates stored within our muscles in the form of glycogen are largely responsible for keeping water inside their cells. Bodybuilders who go on low-carb diets for any appreciable length of time experience a flattening effect on their muscles as the glycogen sheds or releases the water it was bonded to in the muscle cell and hence the muscles "deflate."

Fats: Fats are an important source of fuel that provide energy in low-intensity endurance activities when the more limited glycogen reserves have been depleted. Since certain vitamins are soluble only in fat, it is obvious that fats figure crucially in a well-balanced diet.

Vitamins and minerals: All the various vitamins and minerals are referred to as micronutrients, as they are required in such small quantities each day. Recommended daily intakes of the micronutrients are measured in milligrams and micrograms, as opposed to the grams of the macronutrients. Vitamins and minerals are combined in the body to form the enzymes that serve as catalysts in innumerable physiological processes. If you are consuming a well-balanced diet, you could be getting all the vitamins and minerals you need. If, however, you have any doubt as to whether your diet is balanced, by all means take a general vitamin-mineral supplement.

Water: All of life's complex chemical processes take place in a fluid medium provided by water. The fluidity of our blood and lymph is

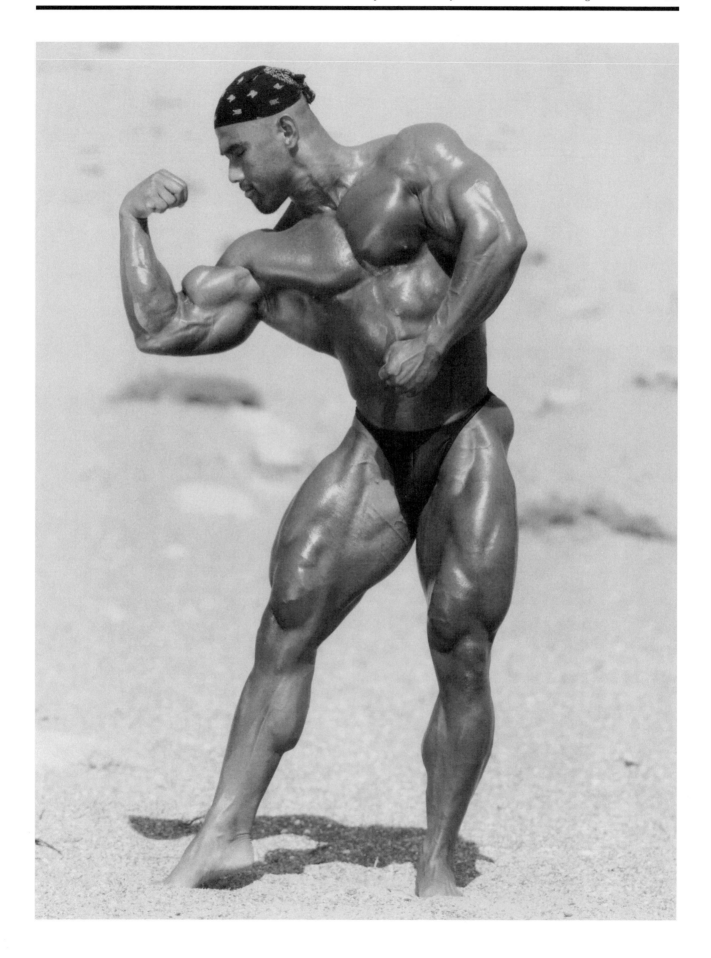

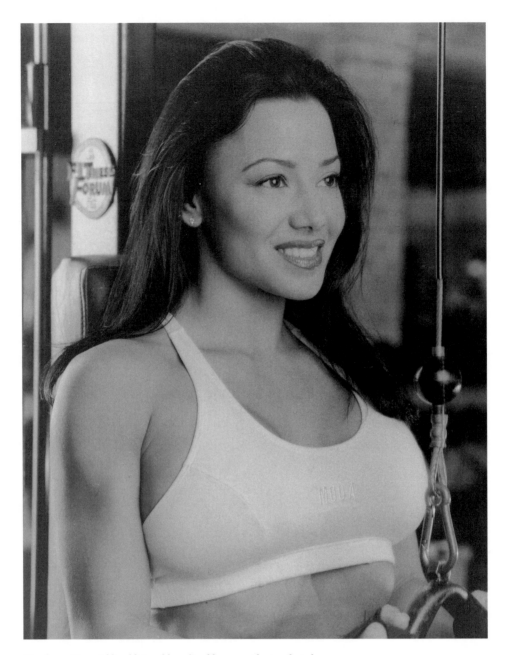

Good nutrition yields additional benefits, like a complexion that glows.

water; it keeps our joints lubricated and helps maintain a constant body temperature; and, not of least importance to the bodybuilder, water is the primary constituent of muscle tissue. Viewed thusly, water could rightly be said to be the most important nutrient for survival as well as for growth. Drinking more water and fluids than thirst dictates is not going to hasten the muscle growth process, however. The body will absorb only what it needs for maintenance and that little bit of growth you might be stimulating on a daily basis—and excrete the rest.

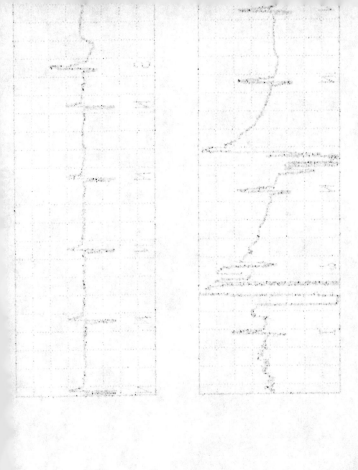

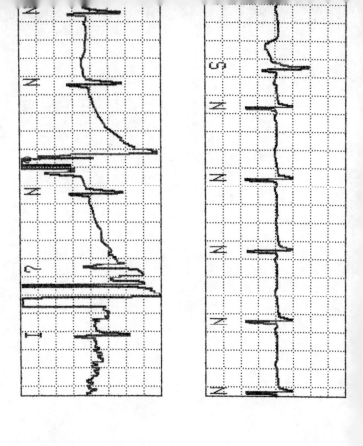

At the beginning of this book we indicated just how slow the muscle growth process typically is, and it's important to consider this in light of the nutritional facts just outlined.

EATING MORE ISN'T THE ANSWER

Eating more food will not cause your muscles to grow at a faster rate. Most of us make the mistake of believing what we read in the muscle magazines—that muscle is made up of protein, so you have to eat lots of it to build bigger muscles. However, as indicated earlier, it just so happens that muscle is comprised of 70 percent water, 22 percent protein, and 6 to 8 percent lipids and inorganic materials. From this we can readily discern that the primary constituent of muscle is not protein—as the magazines that sell protein would have you believe—but water. However, this does not mean that we hasten the muscle growth process by drinking inordinate amounts of water every day, for reasons that we've already touched upon. Unfortunately, you don't have the same impunity with protein because protein contains calories; and when you eat more calories than you need to maintain your existing condition, the excess (apart from that which can be excreted) is stored as fat. And protein can make you just as fat as carbohydrates or fat because excess calories—no matter what their source—make you fat. But such dietary aberrations are simply the result of failing to appreciate just how slow the muscle growth process typically is.

EATING TO BUILD PURE MUSCLE

Let's assume that you're going to be able to apply the principles espoused in this book successfully enough to stimulate 10 pounds of muscle growth over the coming year. Obviously, nutrition must factor into creating those 10 additional pounds—but to what extent? How much food will you have to eat to gain those 10 pounds of pure muscle without adding any body fat?

Well, first of all, you've got to recognize that a pound of muscle tissue contains 600 calories. This is true in all human beings—you or the current Mr. Olympia. If you were to surgically excise a pound of muscle tissue and place it in a device known as a calorimeter, it would give off 600 calories of heat. If you were to gain 10 pounds of muscle mass over the course of one year, you would have to consume 10 × 600 calories or 6,000 calories a year over and above your maintenance need (that is, the amount of calories consumed on a daily basis that is required to maintain your current body weight). You read that correctly, that's 6,000 extra calories a year—not 6,000 extra calories a day, a week, or a month—but 6,000 extra calories *a year*. And eating that amount within a day, a week, or a month will do nothing at all to hasten the muscle growth process. Again, your body has specific nutritional requirements, and any amount above these requirements is eliminated or stored as fat. Still, the

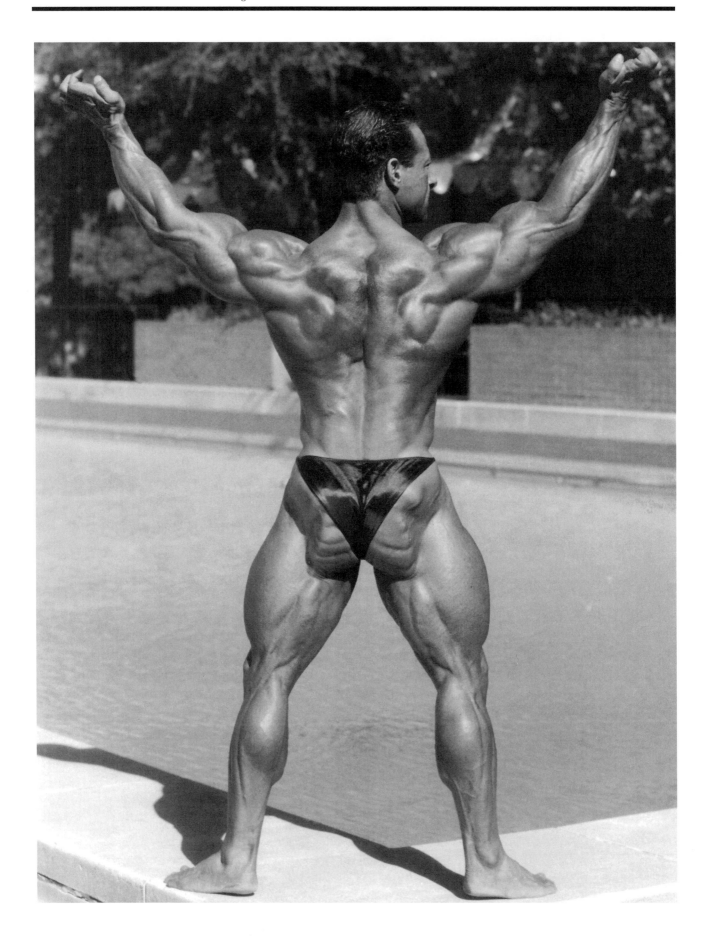

tendency exists for most body-builders to think of their nutritional needs in terms of days. And if we do the math on this, we find that the daily total of extra nutrition required to grow those extra 10 pounds of muscle comes out to approximately 16 extra calories (6,000 calories divided by 365 days) over and above your daily maintenance needs.

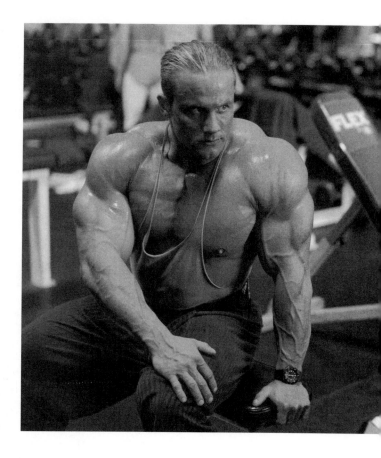

It should be pointed out that the actual process of eating contributes nothing to the growth process. The primary requisite for muscle growth is stimulation—which is done with your Static Contraction Training in the gym. Once this has occurred, nutrition becomes a secondary requisite in that you must provide adequate nutrition to maintain your existing physical mass. Then you've got to provide those 16 calories or so to allow for that tiny bit of extra muscle growth that might be taking place on a daily basis—and we emphasize "might." The fact is that most trainees, regardless of their training preference, already eat more than they need to gain an additional 10 pounds of muscle over the course of a year. If you're not growing muscular mass presently and you're eating sufficiently, then the reason you're not growing is that you're not training with sufficient intensity to stimulate an adaptive muscular response. So, the formula again is: stimulate growth through your high-intensity training and then eat enough to maintain your existing physical mass. Then, to assist in the growth of those additional 10 pounds, you've got to tack on an additional 16 calories a day. If you really want to split hairs, we should acknowledge that the body is not 100 percent efficient, and in fact may need 20 or 30 extra calories in order to yield 16 calories' worth of actual muscle tissue. The point is that you don't need a 2,000-calorie "bodybuilding shake" to get the nutrition you will need.

DETERMINING YOUR MAINTENANCE NEED OF CALORIES

Your maintenance need of calories is simply that: the amount of calories required to maintain your body at your present weight. And the method required to ascertain it is very simple. Every day for five days, write down every

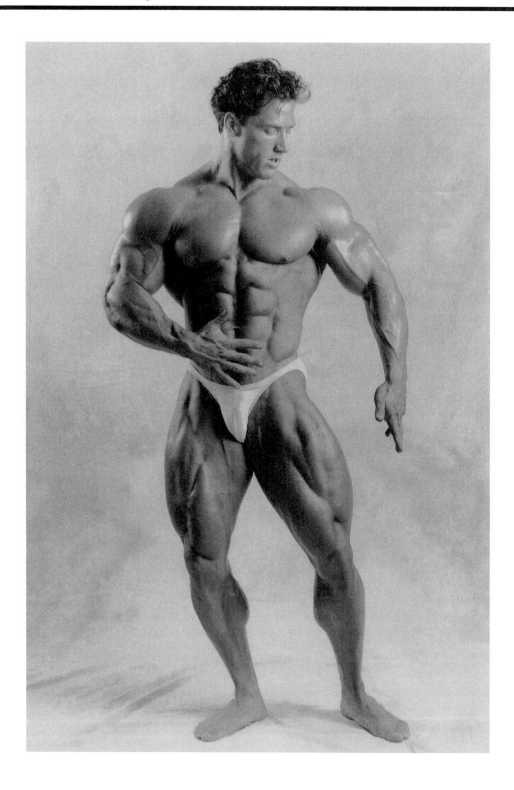

single thing you eat—from the cream you put in your coffee to the dressing you put on your salad. Then, after each day is over, sit down with a calorie-counting book and calculate your total number of calories for that day. After five days, total up your daily caloric totals and divide that number by five. Voila! You've just computed your maintenance need of calories. Here's a hypothetical example of how this might break down:

Monday: You consume a total of 2,500 calories.

Tuesday: You consume a total of 2,700 calories.

Wednesday: It's the middle of the week—a bad week, let us suppose—and you're getting tired and frustrated from your job. You pig out and consume 4,500 calories.

Thursday: You're now feeling guilty for your dietary aberration the day before, and to atone for your misdeed, you only have 1,500 calories.

Friday: Things are back to normal in your life, so your daily intake is 2,500 calories.

When you take these five totals and add them up, the resulting figure comes out to 13,700 calories total for the five days. Now divide this number by five (the number of days), and your resulting daily average is 2,740 calories per day. This is your maintenance need of calories—assuming, of course, that you neither gained nor lost weight during the time you recorded these figures.

This simple method of computing your maintenance need of calories takes into account such diverse and highly individual factors as your basal metabolic rate (BMR) and your voluntary physical activity output. It doesn't even matter how unique or fast your individual metabolism is—it's all taken into account with this formula.

Once your maintenance need of calories has been determined by this method, it becomes a relatively simple procedure to add 16 extra calories a day to your daily average in order to provide that extra nutrition necessary to assist in the growth process, particularly for those extra 10 pounds of pure muscle. With our hypothetical example, this would mean that the daily average caloric intake would be increased from 2,740 to 2,756 per day. And those extra 16 calories can be obtained by simply taking two bites out of an apple!

All of this is simply to underscore the fact that muscle growth is a relatively slow process and that force-feeding yourself hundreds or even thousands of extra calories per day is not going to hasten it at all. In fact, the only thing that force-feeding will succeed in hastening is the size of your waistline.

In conclusion, then, the most important requisite in building muscle mass is stimulating a muscle mass increase through your efforts in the gym. Then stay out of the gym and eat a well-balanced diet that is, perhaps, 16 calories or so higher (per day) than your maintenance need of calories. On the subject of a well-balanced diet, most of our reputable nutritional scientists indicate that a well-balanced diet is comprised of 60 percent carbohydrates, 25 percent protein, and 15 percent fats.

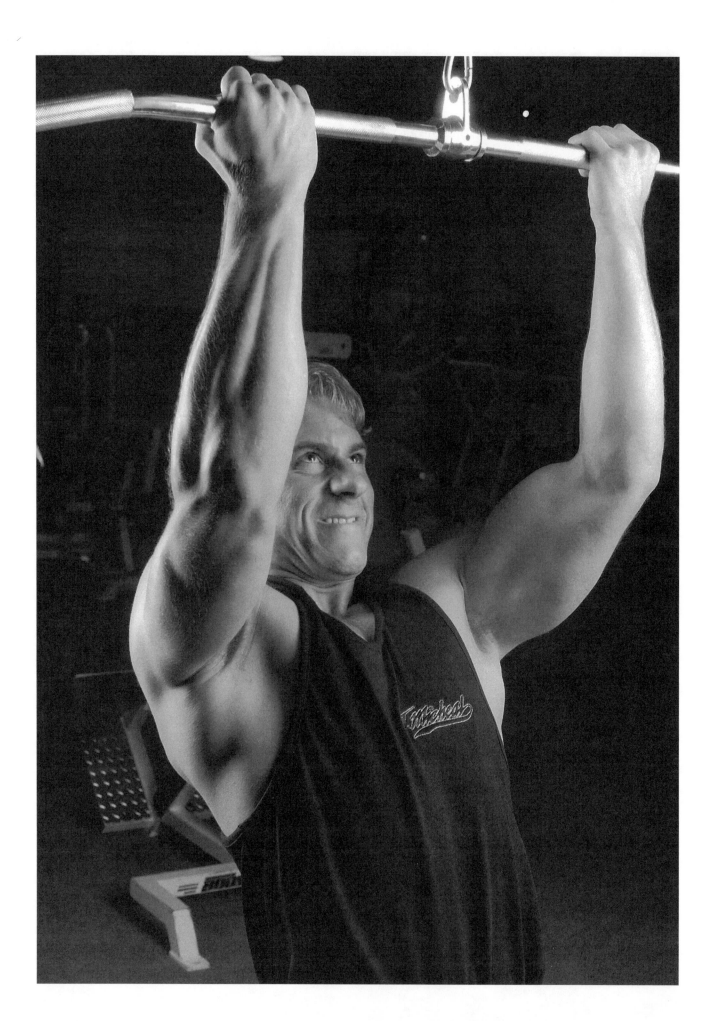

9

Reality Versus Perception in Bodybuilding

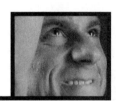

Bodybuilding is a sport that has created some enormous chasms between the truth and what is perceived as the truth. In fact, misrepresentations and flawed logic have marred each of the five critical components of bodybuilding: training, rest, diet, supplementation, and equipment (see the pie charts on page 102). It pays to be mindful of perceptions because you can waste time, money, and progress focusing on elements that are of surprisingly little importance. It's easy to determine what people's perception is of what is important by looking at our mail, E-mail, Internet newsgroup postings, and articles in bodybuilding magazines. Most of the questions and/or articles are on supplements and diet; very few are on training, rest, or equipment.

IMPORTANCE OF TRAINING—
REALITY 40%, PERCEPTION 10%

The fact is that proper training is the only bodybuilding component that can stimulate muscle growth. That's right, the *only* one. So, naturally, we want to know hard facts about exactly what elements of training work best, such as which are the most efficient

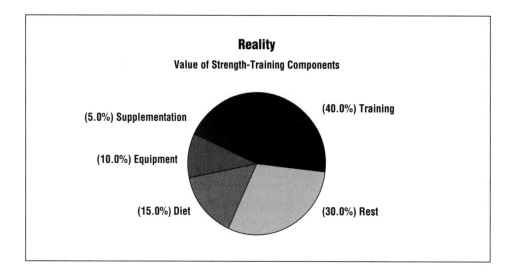

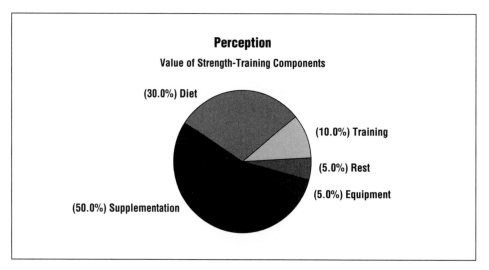

and/or productive exercises. But how many clinical studies on training methodology have you seen undertaken by or printed in bodybuilding magazines? Where is the hard research on the relative intensity of pre-exhaustion versus super sets versus partials? Where are the studies on the effectiveness of dumbbell curls versus cable curls (other than in the book you now hold in your hands)? Such knowledge is not being acquired or properly categorized; instead all training methods are just thrown into the same pot with a sort of moral equivalency so that bodybuilders can just pick whatever piece of equipment isn't being used at the moment and start exercising. If the bodybuilding magazines were doing an honest job in this regard they would be in a constant competition to uncover the latest research in every facet of training and give the "scoop" to their readers. In reality, none of the magazines has ever conducted a single study on training. So most readers perceive training to be unimportant which, in turn, creates little demand for the information.

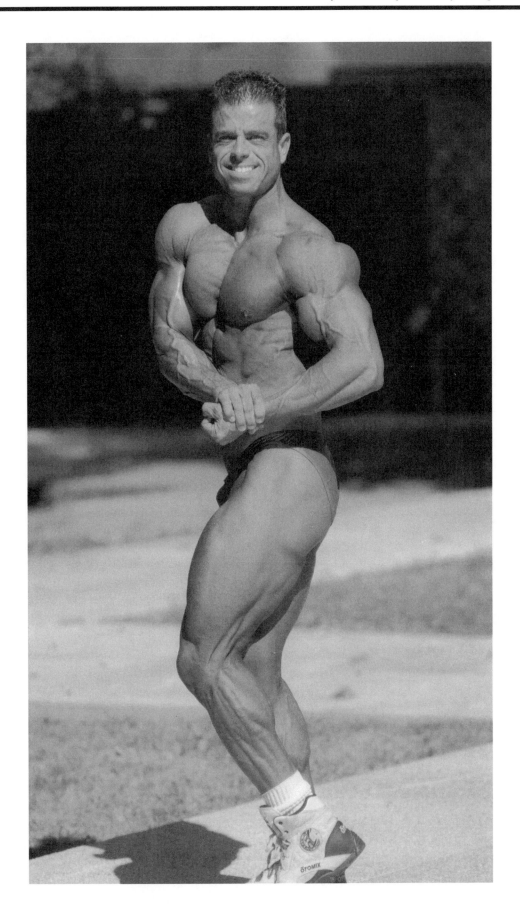

IMPORTANCE OF REST—REALITY 30%, PERCEPTION 5%

People really underestimate the importance of rest. Rest is the most over-looked and misunderstood concept in bodybuilding. Nearly every training system says "Train Monday, Wednesday, and Friday." That's it. No matter who you are or what your circumstance, that's how much rest you should get between workouts. Lately, those who consider themselves more enlightened are saying that you should only work out every three to five days thus giving your body even more rest time. These guys don't get it either. Remember where you heard this: the amount of rest you need is always changing. It's dynamic, not static. When you first start training, you need very little rest time, perhaps as little as 24 hours. Within days, however, your strength will increase to a point where you require 48 hours of rest between workouts. Soon after you will need three or four days of rest. If your strength continues to progress, you will then need five, six, or seven days of rest. Rest requirements are directly related to your strength and the amount of work you perform in a workout. This "rest curve" is ripe for proper scientific study in order to learn how to optimize training. But have you ever seen rest seriously researched and examined in a bodybuilding magazine? The misconception is that everyone needs only 48 hours of rest and this amount will remain the same throughout his training career.

IMPORTANCE OF DIET—REALITY 15%, PERCEPTION 30%

Please understand this: we make no argument against a proper diet. Without a proper diet you will die. However, bodybuilders already have a far above average knowledge of nutrition. Beyond their whole protein, low-fat diet of skinless chicken, rice and beans, and fruits and vegetables, there is little room for improvement. The fact is that once your diet contributes the nutrients your body needs, no more can be done. Extra nutrients are superfluous and just don't help. The extra calories will, however, turn into fat! Spending time trying to find ways to measure the extra muscle building benefits of rice cakes versus wheat bread is not going to yield much in the end.

IMPORTANCE OF SUPPLEMENTATION—
REALITY 5%, PERCEPTION 50%

More misconceptions surround supplementation than any other bodybuilding component. As we just discussed in the previous section on diet, bodybuilders are keenly aware of nutritional considerations. We'll bet that not one bodybuilder in 100 is nutritionally deficient (which would mean that supplementation has an importance of less than 1 percent, but we're feeling generous). For medical reasons you need supplementation when you have some sort of a deficiency. If you are not nutritionally deficient, you *don't* need nutri-

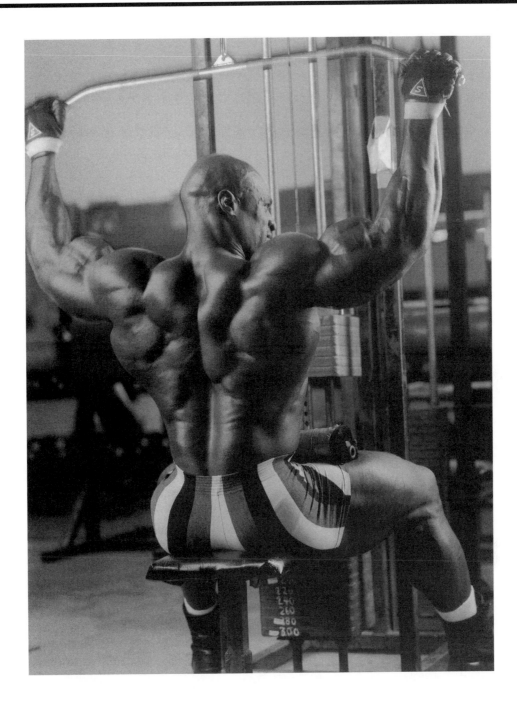

tional supplementation. Of course, no manufacturer of supplements will attest to this. Their ads don't say "Are you tyrosine-deficient? Here's the help you need!" They say "Want to get HUGE? Take tyrosine!" or "Want to get ripped? Take amino acids!" Supplements are sold as "magic bullets" to gullible and/or naive people who want to believe that they will yield such great results without their having to alter such "minor" aspects as training or rest. That supplements are perceived as a very important element is hardly suprising when you consider that supplement ads comprise over 50 percent of the advertising in bodybuilding magazines. The reality is that almost no one needs them.

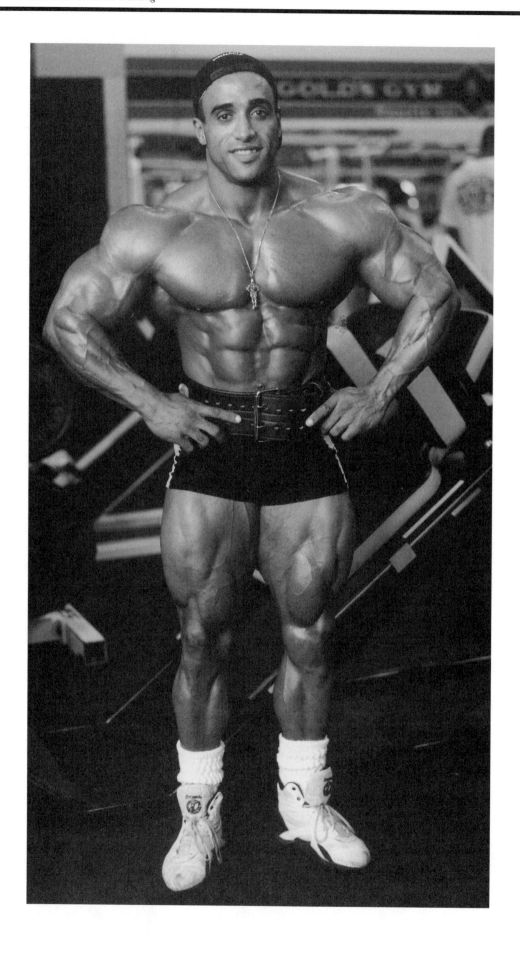

IMPORTANCE OF EQUIPMENT— REALITY 10%, PERCEPTION 5%

Just how important equipment is, is a tough call. On the one hand, lifting a 40-pound bucket of rocks provides the same muscular overload as lifting a 24-karat gold, 40-pound dumbbell. But on the other hand, some manufacturers go to great lengths to design quality equipment that will prevent injury or generate more overload to specific muscle groups. For example, Hammer Strength makes the best grip strength machine of all time. Like all Hammer Strength equipment, the Grip Machine is of top quality and has a smooth-as-glass operation, providing plenty of adjustable overload to guarantee progression for every kind of user up to a mountain gorilla. Another fine product is the Manta Ray device (by Advanced Fitness, Inc.), which clips on any squat bar and prevents cervical disc injury, a great product that could prevent thousands of injuries per year. Such equipment then could obviously be beneficial to bodybuilders; however, innovators of such products go largely unnoticed in bodybuilding magazines. We don't see anybody helping promote them or running comparative articles. Do you know which biceps curl machine provides the most overload or the safest operation—Nautilus? Universal? Hammer Strength? Kaiser?

UNDERSTANDING BODY COMPOSITION

We never realized how misunderstood the concept of body composition was until we spoke to several people in conjunction with the Static Contraction Research Study. One of the "before and after" measurements we had subjects take was their body-fat percentage. What we soon learned was that many people take their body-fat percentage as an isolated number that measures body fat only with the result that in all cases an increase is bad and a decrease is good. The truth is that this is only half of the story.

One person who called us reported his results with obvious disappointment. Along with considerable increases in both static and dynamic strength, his body fat had decreased from 17.6 percent to 14.1 percent but he had gained only four pounds in six weeks, going from 204 pounds to 208 pounds. He was disappointed with such meager "mass" gains and only mildly happy that his body fat had decreased. When we showed him what those numbers really reflected he changed his tune:

Before:	204 pounds @ 17.6 percent body fat = 35.9 pounds of fat and 168.1 pounds of lean muscle
After:	208 pounds @ 14.1 percent body fat = 29.3 pounds of fat and 178.7 pounds of lean muscle
Difference:	a loss of 6.6 pounds of fat and a gain of 10.6 pounds of muscle for a net change of 4.0 pounds on the bathroom scale

Suddenly this guy is over the moon that he gained 10.6 pounds of muscle in just six weeks! The proof had been in front of him all the time, but he just let the numbers sit on the page without ever fully understanding what they represented.

Grade-Six Arithmetic

Here is all you need to know about getting the information you need out of a body-fat measurement. Simply take your body weight (for example, 204 pounds) and multiply it by your body-fat measurement (for example, 17.6 percent). To multiply by a percent just move the decimal point left two spaces so that 17.6 percent becomes .176. (Those fortunate few among you who have single digit body-fat percentages need to insert a zero in front of the number—for example, 8.1 percent becomes .081.) This gives you the weight of fat in your body (204 × .176 = 35.9). Since this is the weight of fat in your body you can subtract this number from your total weight in order to discover your lean mass (204 − 35.9 = 168.1), and you'll find your lean mass is 168.1 pounds. You should remember that this "lean mass" measurement actually represents everything in your body other than fat. That includes bones, blood, organs, and so forth, but since these other parts don't increase significantly from strength training, virtually all of the gains in this number can be attributed to an increase in muscle size and density.

Let's take a look at some common scenarios in order to find the truth about a trainee's progress in the gym:

Scenario #1   Weight goes up 10 pounds (180 pounds to 190 pounds). Body fat goes up 4 percent (15 percent to 19 percent.)

Is this good or bad?

Before: 180 pounds @ 15 percent = 27.0 pounds fat and 153.0 pounds lean muscle

After: 190 pounds @ 19 percent = 36.1 pounds fat and 153.9 pounds of lean muscle

Difference: 9.1 pounds of fat gain and 0.9 pounds of muscle gain

This is a guy who is eating like a pig because somebody told him bodybuilders need to eat huge amounts of food in order to "pack on the mass." The trouble is, the mass he's packing on is fat.

Scenario #2   Weight goes up 10 pounds (120 pounds to 130 pounds). Body fat goes up 4 percent (15 percent to 19 percent). Notice this is the same as Scenario #1 except the trainee is 60 pounds lighter.

Is this good or bad?

Before: 120 pounds @ 15 percent = 18.0 pounds fat and 102.0 pounds lean muscle

After: 130 pounds @ 19 percent = 24.7 pounds fat and 105.3 pounds of lean muscle

Difference: 6.7 pounds of fat gain and 3.3 pounds of muscle gain

This trainee has put on over triple the muscle as #1 and gained less fat. However, his training and diet are still less than ideal since his body fat is increasing.

Scenario #3 Weight goes down 15 pounds (195 pounds to 180 pounds). Body fat goes down 4 percent (15 percent to 11 percent).

Is this good or bad?

Before: 195 pounds @ 15 percent = 29.25 pounds fat and 165.75 pounds lean muscle

After: 180 pounds @ 11 percent = 19.80 pounds fat and 160.20 pounds of lean muscle

Difference: 9.45 pounds of fat loss and 5.55 pounds of muscle loss

This trainee lost both fat and muscle. This is what happens when you diet but do not perform workouts that stimulate new muscle growth. While it is good to lose fifteen unwanted pounds, the fat loss is less likely to remain permanent when it takes nearly 5.5 pounds of muscle with it, thereby reducing the Basal Metabolic Rate by about 300 calories per day (50 calories/pound of muscle). This trainee will have to eat even less now if he wants the fat to stay off.

Scenario #4 Weight goes down 5 pounds (195 pounds to 190 pounds). Body fat goes down 4 percent (15 percent to 11 percent). Note that this is similar to Scenario #3 but with less weight loss.

Is this good or bad?

Before: 195 pounds @ 15 percent = 29.25 pounds fat and 165.75 pounds lean muscle

After: 190 pounds @ 11 percent = 20.90 pounds fat and 169.10 pounds of lean muscle

Difference: 8.35 pounds of fat loss and 3.35 pounds of muscle gain

Notice that this trainee lost nearly as much fat as the trainee in Scenario #3 but without the muscle loss. This is a common and desirable scenario wherein the exercise of productive weight training burns off fat due to the general increase of activity while, at the same time, stimulating new muscle growth. This new muscle will burn more calories to help further reduce fat. This is the third best scenario for a bodybuilder.

Scenario #5 Weight stays the same (190 pounds to 190 pounds). Body fat goes down 4 percent (15 percent to 11 percent).

Is this good or bad?

Before: 190 pounds @ 15 percent = 28.5 pounds fat and 161.5 pounds lean muscle

After: 190 pounds @ 11 percent = 20.9 pounds fat and 169.1 pounds of lean muscle

Difference: 7.6 pounds of fat loss and 7.6 pounds of muscle gain

If this trainee went by the bathroom scale only, he would see zero improvement, get discouraged, and give up. Thanks to body-fat calculations, he can see that he is making great progress. This scenario is second only to Scenario #6 in desirability for a bodybuilder.

Scenario #6   Weight goes up 10 pounds (180 pounds to 190 pounds). Body fat goes down 5 percent (15 percent to 10 percent).

Is this good or bad?

Before: 180 pounds @ 15 percent = 27.0 pounds fat and 153.0 pounds lean muscle

After: 190 pounds @ 10 percent = 19.0 pounds fat and 171.0 pounds of lean muscle

Difference: 8.0 pounds of fat loss and 18.0 pounds of muscle gain

This is what every bodybuilder wants. Notice that although the bathroom scales would indicate only a 10-pound increase, this trainee actually packed on 18 pounds of new muscle!

You can see from the above examples that there are very few pat answers regarding a trainee's weight/body fat gains and/or losses. What might seem at first glance to be progress can actually be backsliding and vice versa. This can lead to another chasm between bodybuilding reality and perception. And that's if you actually know your correct body-fat percentage. With just a bathroom scale you're really blind. How many trainees have given up productive routines, stuck with unproductive routines, spent a fortune on unnessary supplements, or just thrown in the towel because they did not realize the whole truth about their progress?

THE TRUTH ABOUT BODYBUILDING SUPPLEMENTS

The advances in medical science during this century have been astounding. In the previous century people afflicted with epilepsy had holes drilled in their heads to vent the "evil spirits" that occupied their bodies. Death from a tooth infection was quite possible. As science, reason, and rationality accelerated their pace, one discovery or innovation led to several others in a mathematically geometric pattern. Those of us who live in the late 20th century see an acceleration of knowledge and learning that brings new medicines and treatments to the marketplace literally every day. Consequently, today the person with epilepsy need only take one small pill each day to control the disease. The same is true for heart, kidney, or liver problems or nearly anything else you care to name. As a culture we have a belief, supported with plenty of valid evidence, that a pill can solve complex medical problems.

Barely a handful of people in the world know exactly how, for example, lithium controls a bipolar disorder of the brain. The evidence for it is presented in clinical language that is incomprehensible to the majority of us. We are left, however, with the strong impression that technical language is the hallmark of scientific fact. And we trust scientific fact. The trouble is tech-

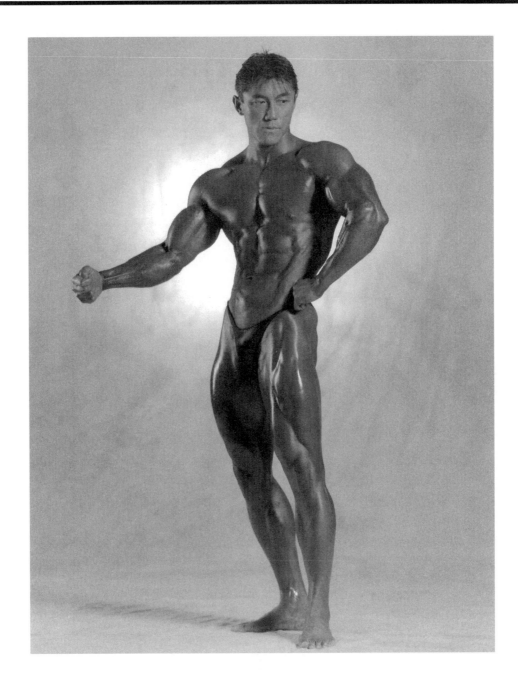

nical language, because most of us do not fully understand it, is a great place to hide unproven premises, mistakes of logic, and outright lies. For example, see how the "ad copy" we created for oranges exploits this technique.

Dartmouth Research Labs' Critical Mass Oranges with Quantum Energy™ only $24.95 each

If you're serious about mass gains you want Critical Mass Oranges with Quantum Energy™. The only oranges certified by Dartmouth Research Labs and guaranteed to provide unsurpassed levels of anti-catabolic nutrients, muscle-cell volumizers, and insulin potentiators to stimulate serious lean mass! How serious? Joe

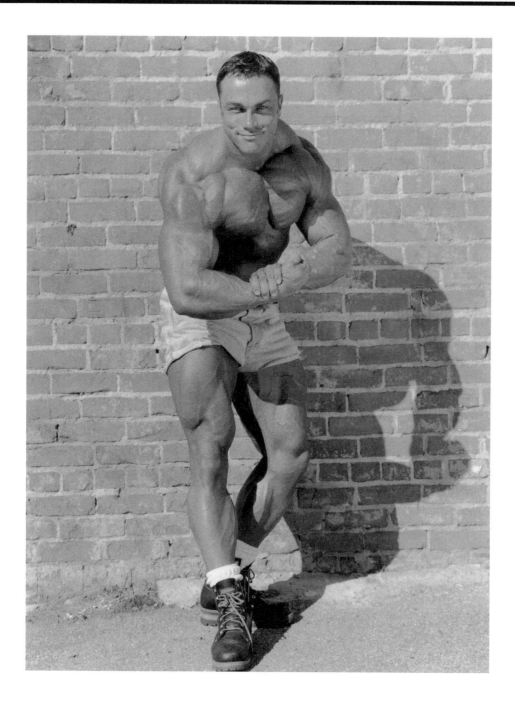

Doaks of Bullroar, Oklahoma, packed on 20 pounds of pure, rock-hard muscle in only one month by incorporating Critical Mass Oranges into his diet. Clinically proven, Quantum Energy™ thermogenic action metabolizes fat and gives you deep cuts and diamond-hard definition! Loaded with a biochemical matrix of nutrients and macronutrients your body needs when performing under stress. Fat-free, lactose-free, no added sugar or sodium. If you want to kick your body into overdrive, don't be fooled by imitators! Get the only oranges certified by Dartmouth Research Labs—Critical Mass Oranges with Quantum Energy™ and pack on the MASS!
(Note: All names and trademarks are fictional.)

Now let's take a look at this literary masterpiece of deception and half-truths. Here is the translation in plain English:

1. Dartmouth Research Labs: Great name but it could be in a guy's basement.
2. Critical Mass Oranges with Quantum Energy™: By law you can give a product a name that suggests the product has certain qualities it really doesn't. For example, you can name a product "Immortality Formula" without it actually containing a formula for immortality. That's good to know when you are looking at a can of "Muscle Builder" in the nutrition store. Similarly with *mass* and *energy* in one product name you might think Einstein's work had a role in the development of Critical Mass Oranges with Quantum Energy™.
3. ". . . Only $24.95 each": Quite expensive for a 15-cent orange but just read what you get!
4. "If you're serious about mass gains . . .": All matter in the universe has mass. When you drink eight ounces of water, you gain eight ounces of mass. Did you think the ad meant muscle mass? They didn't actually say muscle mass, did they?
5. "The only oranges certified by Dartmouth Research Labs . . .": They certify everything they sell and nothing anyone else sells. You pay $24.95 for their own certification—straight from the guy in the basement.
6. ". . . guaranteed to provide unsurpassed levels . . .": *Unsurpassed* means the same levels as everyone else's oranges. No more, no less.
7. ". . . of anti-catabolic nutrients, muscle-cell volumizers, and insulin potentiators . . .": Translation: vitamins, water, and sugar.
8. ". . . to stimulate serious lean mass! . . .": Define *serious*. Here it means almost none. Define *stimulate*. Here it means the water "goes into" your already existing "serious lean" muscles. Of course, it does not and cannot stimulate new muscle growth.
9. Joe Doaks of Bullroar, Oklahoma: Mr. Doaks may or may not exist, and if he does, he's probably a relative of the guy in the basement.
10. ". . . packed on 20 pounds pure, rock-hard muscle in only one month . . .": Maybe, but he also packed on 15 pounds of pure blubbery fat. And you're not Joe Doaks. Joe Doaks is a genetic freak.
11. ". . . by incorporating Critical Mass Oranges into his diet.": Joe also incorporated steroids, growth hormones, clenbuterol, and insulin into his diet. Joe also hadn't trained in over a year and had lost 40 pounds of muscle since being an Olympic powerlifter. Welcome back, Joe.
12. "Clinically proven, Quantum Energy™ thermogenic action . . .": *Thermo* means *heat* in Greek. Oranges have calories which, in physics, is a measurement of heat. So these oranges contain "clinically proven" calories. Wow.

13. "... metabolizes fat and gives you deep cuts and diamond-hard definition!": It takes heat energy to burn fat, or to burn anything else. Whether or not the energy in these oranges is actually used to burn fat depends on how much food you actually eat. The energy could just as well be used to build some more fat for you. *How* deep are the cuts, you ask? One millionth of an inch is all that would be required to make this ad legal. Diamonds can cut glass. Be sure to give us a call when your glutes can cut glass!

14. "Loaded with a biochemical matrix of nutrients and macronutrients ...": Translation: Vitamins and water, mixed together.

15. "... your body needs when performing under stress ...": Your body is always under stress unless you are dead.

16. "Fat-free, lactose-free, no added sugar or sodium.": Same as any other oranges.

17. "If you want to kick your body into overdrive. ...": Your body doesn't have an overdrive.

18. "... don't be fooled by imitators!": Please don't buy the identical oranges for 15 cents.

19. "... and pack on the MASS! ...": About 3 ounces (or whatever the orange weighs) of "MASS," not to be confused with muscle mass.

Get the idea of what technical language can do? And remember this—every word in the above ad is legally true! We could run this ad today in any bodybuilding magazine. Don't believe us? We got every buzzword except the product name for the above ad out of current issues of major bodybuilding magazines!

Use of Psychological Manipulation

We all know that the purpose of advertising is to manipulate the consumer into wanting the product advertised. When we see an ad for a new Buick that features a gorgeous model lying on the fender in an evening dress, we understand that she doesn't come with the Buick. That distinction is blurred when a bodybuilding supplement ad features a male model with a ripped, freaky physique holding up a can of "XYZ Muscle Builder." Some people are naturally going to assume that the advertised product will build that kind of physique. But it won't. It can't.

Here is a fact that you must never forget: There is no food, food supplement, or even a drug that can, by itself, put muscle on your body. Muscle only grows as a result of direct stimulation in the form of overload. You have to make your muscles work if you want them to grow bigger and stronger. Even if you take steroids and testosterone and then just sit on the sofa all day, the drugs will not create new muscle. (Before you think we're promoting drugs in bodybuilding, read Drugs in Bodybuilding at the end of this chapter.) In the case of foods and nutritional supplements, they only support the growth of muscle that has been stimulated by work—they cannot generate extra muscle because of their "unique blend" or "patented matrix" or "scientific formula." Not convinced? Here is the fine print taken directly from the label of a top-selling supplement of a major company:

> *As with all supplements, use of this product will not promote faster or greater muscular gains. This product is, however, a nutritious low-fat food supplement which, like other foods, provides nutritional support for weight-training athletes.*

Let's look at that first sentence with some emphasis added: "As with ALL supplements, use of this product will NOT promote FASTER OR GREATER muscular gains." So here is how the conversation should go when you go into the nutrition store to buy this product:

> You: *Hi, I'm a bodybuilder and I'm looking for something that will help me put on more muscle.*
>
> Clerk: *OK! Well, we've got all kinds of mass builders. How about this Brand X? It's only $13!*
>
> You: *Great. Will it promote greater muscular gains? I mean, will I get more muscle than I would without it?*
>
> Clerk: *No.*
>
> You: *Well, will the muscle I am going to get develop any faster because I use this?*
>
> Clerk: *No.*
>
> You: *Well, if I don't get extra muscle growth or faster muscle growth, why should I take it?*
>
> Clerk: *Ahh . . . it tastes less chalky than many others, and if you eat this, you won't have to eat regular, tasty food.*
>
> You: *But I like regular, tasty food.*
>
> Clerk: *(looking at label) But this has a biopolymeric protein complex, crystalline fructose complex carbohydrate system.*
>
> You: *So does regular, tasty food. Do you have one supplement in this store that will put more muscle on me?*
>
> Clerk: *No.*
>
> You: *Thanks. Good-bye.*

So why is anyone paying $13 a can for this product? No extra muscle, no faster muscle. Moreover, the suggested use for Brand X requires about 10 cans a month for a total of $130. And how about the statement, "As with all supplements . . ."? If you were selling a successful product wouldn't you sue the Brand X company for making a statement that basically says your product won't promote faster or greater muscular gains either? They haven't. The Brand X company is telling the truth when it says, "As with ALL supplements, use of this product will not promote faster or greater muscular gains." So the supplement companies have to use psychological tricks like having a huge, steroid monster hold up a product so you'll think that's how he got so big. Or they appeal to your insecurity; an old muscle magazine ad that offered time payments for equipment used to say, "Now being short of cash is no excuse for puny weakness." "Puny weakness?" That's a psychological kick in the groin to an 18-year-old ectomorph.

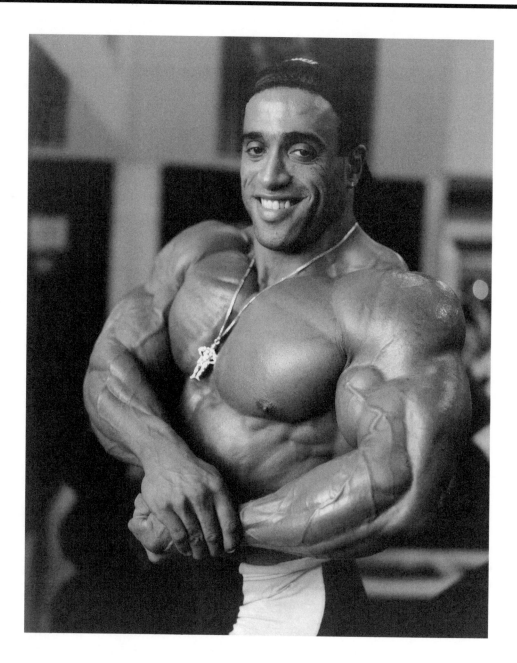

Truth in Packaging

There is a legal flaw in the advertising and packaging of nutritional supplements. The Federal Trade Commission (FTC) has jurisdiction over advertising claims. The FTC generally responds only to consumer complaints, and there must be a lot of them before the FTC will investigate a company making false advertising claims. An ad can run for months, even years, before enough people have complained in order for the FTC to approach the offending company. The FTC will demand that the supplement company pull the ad. The company complies and then has its advertising department simply create a new ad that says something different—still misleading, but different.

In contrast, the consequences for making false medical claims on a product package can be severe. Jurisdiction over packaging labels belongs to the

Food and Drug Administration (FDA), which will assess an offending company with serious penalties of large fines or possible imprisonment. Repeat offenders can find themselves doing serious jail time. Consequently, there are few companies indeed that will make fantastic claims on their product labels.

Go into any nutrition store and look at labels. Products carry names (names are not regulated) like "Fat Metabolizer," "Thyroid Support," "Nutra Trim," and "Thyro-Boost." But when you read the label, you'll never find any copy saying the product will actually increase fat loss or thyroid function. Such claims have to be supported with objective, clinical proof. Supplement companies thus choose product names that will imply that a product will help you achieve certain results (such as to increase fat loss). What you will find on product labels are such noncommital claims as "made with all natural ingredients," "certified pure by independent laboratory analysis," " free of animal products," "maximum potency," and on and on. There is always a list of the product's ingredients as well, but never any statements of what medical problem the supplement is alleged to help or cure. Ads, however, nearly always mention specific medical problems (obesity, prostate, thyroid, and so on) or bodybuilding goals (such as getting ripped or packing on muscle), but the actual product labels (despite a product's name) merely list ingredients. Now you know why.

Your Loss Is Their Gain

The false premise in nearly all of the nutritional supplement hype is the assumption that your body is not getting adequate amino acids, vitamins, minerals, bee pollen, or whatever. Advertisers, for example, claim that amino acids are essential in the muscle-building process. Gulping down $20 a day in protein, however, will not help build more muscle. When you exercise sufficiently to trigger the growth of, say, three ounces of new muscle growth, your body uses the ingredients it needs to make that three ounces of muscle. Your consuming more ingredients (nutrients) will not result in two pounds of muscle growth. The extra nutrients will either increase your body fat or be eliminated. Either way, what you will gain from supplements is expensive fat or urine.

Speaking of expense, we purchased 20 supplemental products from a nutrition store and analyzed the labels. We looked at the cost per serving and the cost per month of maintaining the suggested servings and found that these costs vary greatly from one supplement manufacturer to another. For example, one brand of creatine monohydrate says to take three to five capsules one hour before a workout. Each capsule contains 725 mg of creatine monohydrate. So a big guy taking five capsules for a total of 3,625 mg and working out three times a week will consume about 60 capsules a month. We bought a pack of 12 for $4.99 so the monthly cost would be about $25. Another brand, however, recommends a "maintenance dose" for persons over 225 pounds of 10,000 mg every day. Over a month that's 635 percent more than the first brand's recommendation. One of us managed to get seven days' worth out of a bottle costing $23.95. That makes a cost per month of over $102. By the way, five days of an initial "loading dose" will cost you another 50 bucks!

Such was the case for creatine monohydrate. What about metabolic optimizers, complete foods, ripped enhancers, and amino acids, to name a few?

Well, if you took the recommended servings of all the products we bought you'd be shelling out 1,650 bucks a month. That's 20 grand a year of take-home pay! But the money spent will result in huge, ripped muscles, right? Wrong.

Who Can You Believe?

So, do any supplements have a positive effect? With the hundreds of products on the market you'd think that there would be one or two good ones. That's possible. But how can you trust a company that lies in its ads, misuses terms like *anabolic* and *steroid replacement*, tells only half the story of related clinical studies, uses steroid monsters to imply impossible results, or charges you 400 percent more than a competitor for the same chemical compound? You just can't trust them. And if you insist on running your own "clinical trial," ask yourself this question: "What is a pound of muscle worth to me?" Hypothetically, if a year's worth of the top-selling supplement at a cost of $4,000 a year, along with your weight training, added an extra 10 pounds of muscle to your body, you would be paying over $400 for each pound gained! If that's acceptable to you, bon appétit.

Supplements Are Just Food

Understand this: nutritional supplements are foods. That's it! You can buy a bag of carrots, or you can buy a bottle of powdered carrot extract, but either way, it's just food. Remember our parody advertisement for the Dartmouth Research Labs Critical Mass Oranges with Quantum Energy™? The whole point is that you can buy a certain kind of food, or you can buy expensive supplements that have the same chemical constituents as that food. Either way all you are getting is the food, in this case, oranges.

For example, if we told you that eating a lot of apples would "really pack on the muscle," would you believe it? Probably not. Most of us have eaten apples all our lives, and no one has made a connection between eating apples and developing muscle mass. But an apple has thousands of different chemicals that make up its characteristics. So suppose we took one of those chemicals, say pectin, and started telling you, via colorful, well-worded magazine ads, that in order to get X milligrams of pectin, which is "vital" for building muscle, you'd have to eat 30 apples a day. To get all the muscle building benefits of X milligrams of pectin, you shouldn't eat all those high-calorie apples; instead just take these pectin tablets! Would you write us a letter asking if this new pectin supplement really works? Save yourself a stamp. All supplements are just food.

Half-Truths Build an Industry

One of us spoke to an insider in the supplement business who said that the initial studies on creatine monohydrate were performed with vegetarian test subjects. Let's examine the study. Creatine monohydrate is a compound found, in highest concentrations, in red meat and is used by the muscles during exercise. People who never eat red meat are quite likely to be creatine-deficient. So a group of subjects who are creatine-deficient and fed megadoses of creatine are bound to manifest improved muscle function (strength and mass gains) compared to another control group of vegetarians that remained creatine-deficient. (Moreover, once muscles are saturated with creatine monohydrate, no further gains are possible.) I happen to eat red meat; you probably do also. So we shouldn't expect any benefits from taking creatine. Does the advertising say that? Does it say, "Attention vegetarians, you may be creatine-deficient?" No. The ad says *everyone* should take the product and keep taking it 365 days a year.

The Long-Term Effects

And there is a much larger question that needs to be answered. What are the long-term effects of taking certain supplements? Are people who take supplements out of concern for their health unknowingly running the risk of developing serious side effects in the future? The consumption of red meat has been linked, by reliable medical studies, to various kinds of cancer, although it is unclear exactly what the connection is between red meat and cancer. Perhaps, just perhaps, it's the creatine monohydrate, which, as we noted above, is found in red meat. Some "recommended doses" of the supplement for creatine monohydrate are the equivalent of five pounds of red meat per day! But what are the long-term health effects of eating five pounds of red meat a day, regardless of the form in which it's eaten? Does anyone know? The companies selling this supplement don't seem to care, in our opinion, whether the long-term consumption of such unnaturally huge quantities of their product will cause cancer. And who will ever perform such a study? Since Americans don't eat five pounds of meat a day, it's hardly a pressing question for responsible scientists. They also won't be testing the long-term effects of eating two dozen peaches, ten loaves of bread, or twenty bananas per day. After all, outside of bodybuilding, who'd consume food or food supplements in those quantities?

Melatonin is another popular supplement that is heavily advertised on radio and in print. Melatonin is not targeted to bodybuilders; it's touted for anyone who is having trouble sleeping. Melatonin is a hormone and the supplemental use of it is predicated on a common bit of illogic used in the nutrition business. As you grow older, the illogic goes, the amount of melatonin your body produces decreases; therefore, if you artificially increase the level of melatonin when you are older, you'll feel young again. But does anyone examine what the long-term effects of artificially high levels of this hormone can do, particularly when we are older? Perhaps there is a reason that millions of years of human evolution have come to reduce melatonin as we age. Maybe we should leave it alone. Moreover, the logic is flawed. When we were 18, we had more pimples than we do now in our thirties. Will artificially adding pimples, or the oils and hormones that caused them, make our bodies feel 18 again? Is it time for pimple implants? Can supplement companies get the clock to run backward by duplicating two or three hormone or enzyme levels out of the thousands that make up our metabolism? Did Ponce de Leon find the Fountain of Youth? Well, neither has anyone else.

Here's an even more overt example of how supplement companies fail to notify the public of the possible negative side effects of their products. Recently it was reported that the common nutritional supplement chromium picolinate when introduced into cells, manifested DNA damage of the kind associated with cancer. Admittedly, these were preliminary studies done on cells only, not on animals or humans. At any rate, the type of cell damage caused by chromium picolinate was the same kind caused by known carcinogens. If we ran a company selling a product that we thought was safe and then found out about a study like that, we'd pull the product off the shelves as fast as we could and wait for more conclusive studies to be conducted. Wouldn't you? Yet did you see any urgent notices in the bodybuilding magazines? Did you see any supplement companies urging caution? We didn't. They still offer chromium picolinate as a "muscle builder" and "fat reducer." People might be buying a product out of concern for their good health only to have that very product take their health away. Permanently.

It's Trademarked and Patented

Here's something you'll see in virtually every supplement ad. Remember, supplements are just food and you cannot patent a food. If you want to sell someone garlic by telling him it will make him feel 20 years younger, you have to find a way to get him to buy your garlic, not the stuff at the grocery store which costs far less. So you give it a name like Nature's Divine Garden Garlic and then trademark the name. Next you grind it into a powder and put it inside a caplet. The powder-in-a-caplet idea can now be patented. The sole purpose

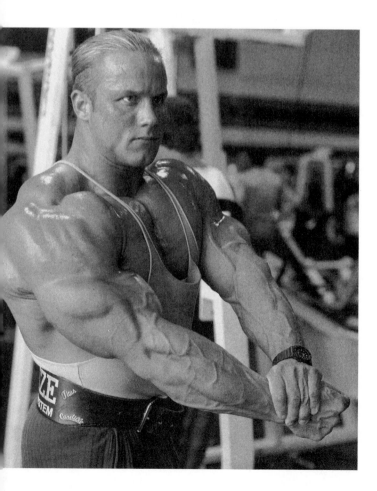

is to give the impression that your garlic (or other supplement) is "so effective it's patented" and is in some way different from everybody else's. But there is no difference. The Law of Constant Composition of Matter states that any given compound always contains the same elements mixed in the same proportions, measured according to their mass. Table salt consists of sodium and chloride and nothing else. All salt is the same. Add a little extra sodium or chloride, and it's no longer salt; it's something else. The same goes for creatine monohydrate—it's all the same. Using various advertising gimmicks, companies fight for brand loyalty by urging you to buy their product because it's somehow unique, be it in powdered form, or with a pH coating, or because it's "all natural" (a meaningless term since lead, arsenic, and salmonella are also "all natural"). But it all amounts to smoke and mirrors.

Supplement du Jour

If you want more evidence that none of these advertised products puts muscle on or takes fat off your body, take a look at some 15- or 20-year old bodybuilding magazines. We remember when everyone was talking about orchic. Orchic was pulverized bull testicles; if you really wanted to pack on the mass, it was the stuff to buy, or so the advertisements said. Where is it today? Nowhere, because it doesn't work. Likewise, is anyone in your gym swearing that milk and egg protein is responsible for his huge muscle development? Nope. But a few years ago it was flying off the shelves as the protein you had to have, sort of like creatine is today. Remember colostrum? That's the substance created in lactating mammals for a short period of time before breast milk is produced. The hypothesis went like this; newborn babies grow at a tremendous rate, and they all consume colostrum. Therefore, a 200-pound adult male who consumes colostrum will grow at a tremendous rate as well. Brilliant. Bodybuilders believed it. (Psst! Want to buy some Gerber baby food at $10 a bottle?)

Where are these products today? They're gone because they don't work. But they will be replaced with other compounds with three- or four-letter names (such as OMT, PAS, IABS) that hopeful bodybuilders will buy with dreams of "packing on the muscle" or "burning off the fat" dancing through their heads.

Let the Buyer Beware

Recently, one of us spoke with a person who makes her living, indirectly, in the nutritional supplement business. On the subject of the possible medical harm caused by long-term use of supplements her principle defense was "Let the buyer beware." She maintained that people need to be up-to-date on studies like the one on chromium picolinate and its possible link to cancer. Her thinking was that people need to try different products to discover "what works for them" and should be aware of the possible harm or side effects of the various nutritional supplements.

Would she take the same approach to children's cough syrup? For example, suppose a major pharmaceutical manufacturer of a children's cough syrup came to know that use of the product could cause leukemia in children. Is it ethical for them to keep it on the market? Should the consumer just try various products to discover "what works" for his kid and all the while keep up-to-date on all the recent clinical studies on cough syrup? Should the consumer be expected to know about a small study done, say, in Helsinki, Finland? If his kid dies from taking the cough syrup, is it "tough beans? He should have been more aware of the related clinical studies!" Should that logic apply to all drugs and their applications? It's ludicrous. There should be legal liability for any company that markets a product that it knows could be dangerous to the user.

The Real Challenge

The two most common complaints that physicians hear from their patients is a lack of energy and a desire to lose weight. Multibillion-dollar, international pharmaceutical companies that develop life-saving products like heart medications and sophisticated antibiotics are dedicating huge financial resources to manufacture a drug that will give people more energy and/or help them remove body fat. Occasionally they edge closer to a solution by finding a piece of the puzzle, which leads to tremendous interest on Wall Street and widespread reporting on television networks and in newspapers everywhere. The first company to develop a pill that removes fat from the human body will make billions of dollars almost overnight. The market for such a drug is worldwide, at least in countries with enough food and wealth to create fat people. Pharmaceutical companies, and their shareholders, are keenly aware that they are in a race with each other and cannot ignore any drug, food, or plant that shows promise. Given that, isn't it highly unlikely that some unheard of company with no reputation for innovation has developed a "fat metabolizer," which is only available from a post office box in Biloxi, Mississippi?

Energy in a tablet? A fat-reducing pill? Don't believe it until you read about such a drug in the *New York Times, Newsweek,* and *Journal of the American Medical Association* and hear Dan Rather and Tom Brokaw reporting it.

Take This! It Works!

The number-one secret weapon of every nutritional supplement manufacturer is the placebo effect. The placebo effect in medicine is not only well documented but also startling in its magnitude. For example, say that patients with abnormal heart conditions are given a placebo said to be an experimental new drug proven effective at treating their kind of heart condition. With that knowledge and nothing else, up to a whopping 40 percent of patients on the placebo will actually manifest improved cardiac function! How can the mind effect an autonomic function such as a heartbeat? This amazing human capacity makes it difficult to test the effects of a drug, or a food supplement, without having the test subject's frame of mind influence the results in some way.

Knowing this, you can guess what happens to certain people who hear about a new bodybuilding supplement from a friend who claims that it enabled him to put 40 pounds on his bench press and gain five pounds in one month. People naturally tend to believe a friend's endorsement of a product over an ad in a magazine or the glib words of a salesclerk. So they buy the stuff, take it, and head for the gym full of enthusiasm and vigor. They tear through their normally boring workout with passion and, not surprisingly, set a personal best or two in the process. That extra effort *will* most likely stimulate some new muscle growth (remember, intensity and progressive overload). During their next visit at the gym, they really are stronger, and have all the psychological motivation of the last workout, so they set some more personal records! Wow! The understandable conclusion is "This stuff really does work!" Their next step will be to tell one or two of their friends about the supplement so they can get the benefit, too. The cycle repeats itself. And that's the mechanism that keeps the nutritional supplement business alive. In fact, the supplement has not brought about these amazing results. What's really working is the power of suggestion and the placebo effect. The increased training intensity put the new muscle on these people, not the chemical action of the supplement.

This phenomenon can feed the manufacturer with hundreds, even thousands, of earnest testimonial letters from customers who believe that the product really worked. There is one problem for the manufacturers, however. The placebo effect only works on 10 to 40 percent of people, so the word of mouth eventually diminishes. It's a mathematical law. Perhaps two people out of ten who buy the product will recommend it to a friend; of those few new people only 20 percent will recommend it to their friends and so on. The customer base keeps diminishing. The manufacturer's only defense is to bring in new customers through advertising, but that too reaches the point of diminishing returns. It's cheaper to announce an all-new wonder supplement and start everyone all over again. This is why the supplement companies are constantly introducing new products. None of their products ever endures because they don't work, and eventually the customers abandon the product.

Can't You Say Anything Good About Supplements?

Are there any positive aspects of nutritional supplements? Yes, one. Bodybuilders who are trying to reduce body fat by decreasing their caloric intake to the absolute minimum can take certain supplements, which will provide them with important nutrients in a low-calorie form. It's hard to get a balanced diet when your caloric intake gets below about 1,200 calories per day. If you eat enough regular, tasty food to get all the nutrients you need, you'll end up eating too many calories. So you're forced to get your nutrients from awful-tasting supplements while on the low-calorie diet.

Somewhere along the line illogic got applied and people began to think that in order to get the huge muscles of pro bodybuilders, they had to consume the strange nutritional "milkshakes" that the bodybuilders were drinking. The "milkshakes" were just low-calorie drinks loaded with nutrients that the old-timers took while on a diet to burn off every scrap of body fat before a contest. The rest of the year—when they were actually gaining muscle—they ate like pigs. There never was anything in those "milkshakes" that added muscle, and there still isn't.

Most people believe that the heyday of snake oil sales was at the turn of the century. A picture comes to mind of a fast-talking huckster standing at the back of a wagon telling the gathered crowd that his Doc Wilson's Elixir cures arthritis, baldness, canker sores, coughs, colds, and lethargy. Today Doc Wilson's progeny have thousands of retail outlets, catalog suppliers, trade shows, full-time Washington lobbyists, and political action committees. And they are still making unproven claims.

DRUGS IN BODYBUILDING

Remember the days when someone would see a big guy in the gym and say, "He must be on steroids." Well, steroids don't even begin to tell the story these days. Take all the steroids your body can tolerate and you won't even qualify for an amateur contest, let alone win. Amateur and professional bodybuilders today take over 35 different drugs like diuretics, amphetamines, blood platelet aggregation inhibitors, thyroid hormones, blood viscosity conditioners, estrogen antagonists, and on and on. Don't forget all of these are taken in addition to the bedrock of testosterone, human growth hormone, insulin, and a grab bag of your garden-variety steroids. Still have a lagging body part? Just inject some esiclene directly into the muscle, and it will swell up like it was hit with a baseball bat. And it stays that way right through judging.

It's well known in the sport that drugs are an everyday fact of life in bodybuilding. Once co-author John Little asked a pro what he took in the off-season. Here is the list exactly transcribed from the athlete's handwritten note.

Off-season
600 mg. Cyp. every other day
300 mg. testosterone suspension every other day
10 dianabol every day
4 anadrol every day
10–20 clenbuterol every day
1 oz. of marijuana per week

This is nonstop—no time off.

6 weeks out [6 weeks from contest]
1 parabolin + 1 primo depo T every other day
3 cc testosterone suspension every other day
50 mg. of halotestin
2 fastin a day
20–25 clenbuterol a day
percadan as needed
1 oz. of marijuana per week

Quite a picture of the healthy fitness lifestyle, huh? This list was just off the top of his head so he can be forgiven for leaving off a few essentials. Thinking of trying this yourself? Don't. Take this many drugs, and you won't wake up tomorrow morning. It takes years to build up a tolerance to this kind of dosage; some bodybuilders never do, so they can't compete in this sport. Twenty-five clenbuterol a day! Next time you take a vitamin, pour 25 of them into your hand and imagine that's your daily overdose of only one of the ten illegal drugs you're taking. Many of the others have to be injected.

Have you ever read some wordy defense of steroid use in a bodybuilding magazine or book quoting medical studies that showed no harmful side effects? When responsible physicians do clinical studies they don't give subjects 20 times the recommended dosage, and they don't keep them on a drug for five years. Moreover, no doctor (with the exception of the Nazi Joseph Mengele) would put a patient on an overdose of 15 or 20 drugs for years on end. Side effects? There never will be clinical studies to document the side effects of such drug "cocktails." Nevertheless, your choice of cancer, leukemia, kidney failure, liver damage, testicular atrophy, sterility, and chromosome damage is virtually inevitable.

What do the official bodybuilding contest rules say? The IFBB (International Federation of Bodybuilding) rules say that drugs are illegal and that drug tests will be conducted. They aren't. How does that make the sport look? About like pro wrestling—a carnival sideshow. By contrast, imagine if the New York Yankees put 14 men on the field during every game, just blatantly cheated. But the umpires, the managers, the players on the other team, the broadcast announcers, the sportswriters, and the fans all said nothing. Nobody yelled, "They're cheating. They've got more men on the field than the rules allow." The game of baseball would be burlesqued and corrupted, the fans would lose interest, and the sport would lose all credibility in the eyes of serious pro athletes. Sound familiar?

Bodybuilding is killing its own market, eating its young. And speaking of the young, what happens when new people get interested in bodybuilding, perhaps as a way to increase their strength for another sport? They pick up one of the magazines and see the guy on the cover, the guys in the ads, the guys in the gossip columns, and the guys in every contest—all huge, ripped, freaky, mass monsters. And that monster, my friends, becomes the standard in their eyes, the standard built on $25,000 to $50,000 worth of black-market drugs a year. That's the standard to which they aspire, one which is very likely to end in medical disaster in either the short-term or long-term future. If they're lucky, they never find out that they're not achieving their aspirations because they're not on the juice. Lucky because they just drop out of the sport and look for something else—a far better fate than "going for the gold" in pro bodybuilding.

A few pro bodybuilders die and countless others are narrowly saved from death by the quick action of fellow competitors and hospital emergency physicians. How does the world of pro bodybuilding react? It just opens up another can of bodybuilders. And the cruelest irony is that the bodybuilders hate being on drugs! All of them. They know they're being exploited and pressured so that the big players—the supplement companies and promoters—in the sport can make more money off them due to their freaky physiques. They're told "Win this contest and you'll get a contract to hold up cans of XYZ Supplements in all our magazine ads."

Imagine being a serious athlete in a sport that you love, having natural ability and superior genetics, having your mom and dad and friends encouraging you, busting your butt in the gym to squeeze every shred of potential from your body, and watching your diet like a supermodel only to lose to a guy who has a drug connection to a new growth hormone straight from a pharmaceutical company in Switzerland. Such is a typical situation in professional bodybuilding. The guy who wins gets a contract to lie about some creatine monohydrate or the "supplement du jour," which he's never taken in his life. The loser drops out of the sport. A few years later the champ does too. And 10 years later neither of them has anything to remind him of the old days except his regular trips to the clinic to get his kidney tumors looked at by his oncologist.

That's the reality of what drug use has done to bodybuilding.

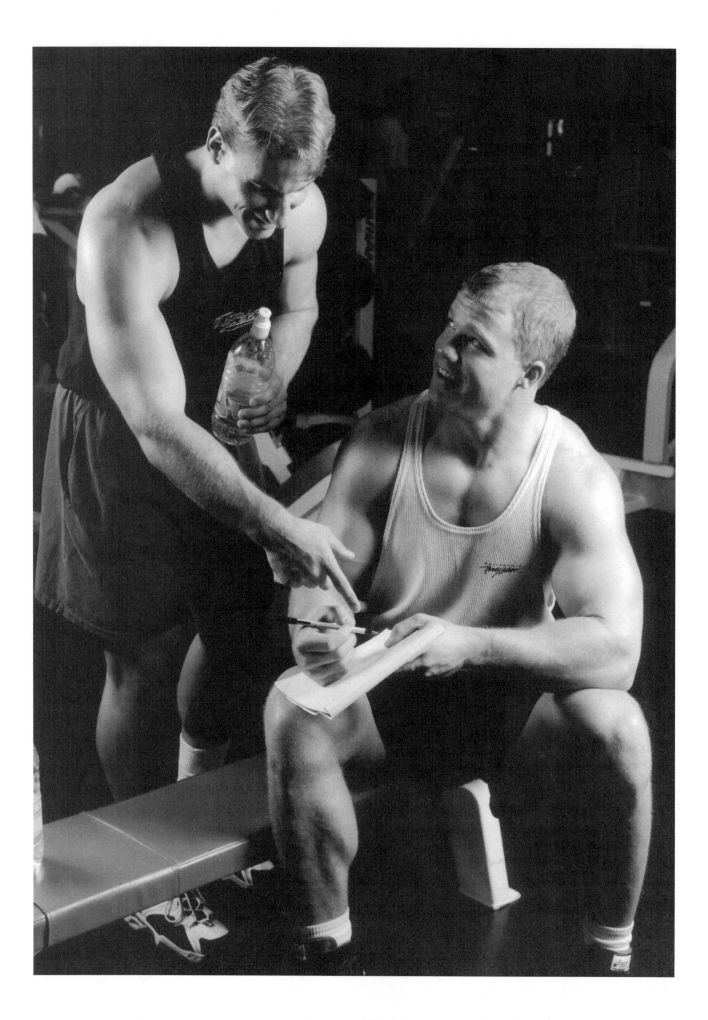

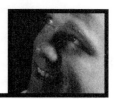

Questions and Answers

10

Question: What is the number-one mistake people make in Static Contraction Training?

Answer: They choose weights that are too light. In every case where we have supervised a workout, trainees are oblivious to how much strength they have in their strong range. For example, in our study with golfers, the women typically used 20 to 30 pounds on the leg extension machine when doing conventional training. Yet in their first static contraction workout they were holding 100 pounds, and six weeks later they were holding over 200 pounds! These were diminutive, middle-aged ladies who belonged to a private club and golfed for recreation; they were not bodybuilders.

The authors perform the same exercise with 700 pounds. (Actually 350 pounds, one leg at a time.) One of us performs 1,000-pound shrugs, and the other is two workouts away from that weight. It is very common for leg press weights to approach or exceed 2,000 pounds in very strong men.

Despite these facts, we still get the occasional letter from someone who says, "I could full-range bench 200 pounds. After two months of Static Contraction Training, I worked up to a 300-pound static hold, but when I checked my full-range bench press it was still just 200. Static Contraction Training didn't work for

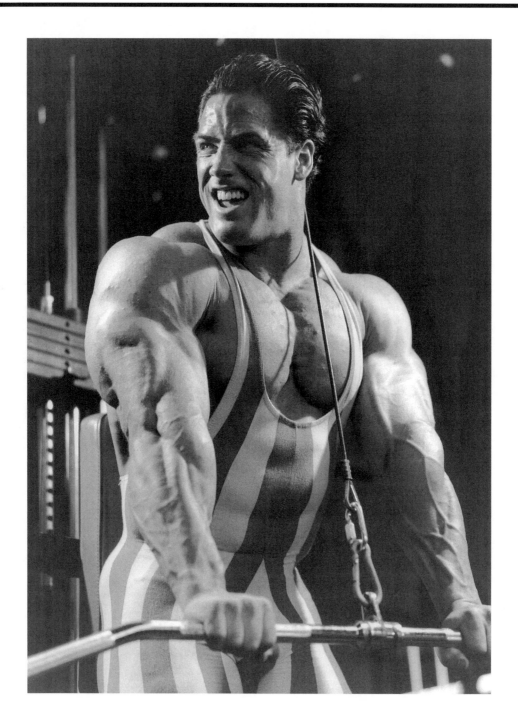

me." The truth is, he didn't work for it. If a person can full-range bench 200, he should be doing static holds with 300 on the first day. In two months he should be in the 500 to 600 pound range . . . that stimulates enormous growth!

Question: What is the number-two mistake people make?

Answer: They work out too often or augment their training with other workouts. This is a tough one to get across to people. Rest is very important!

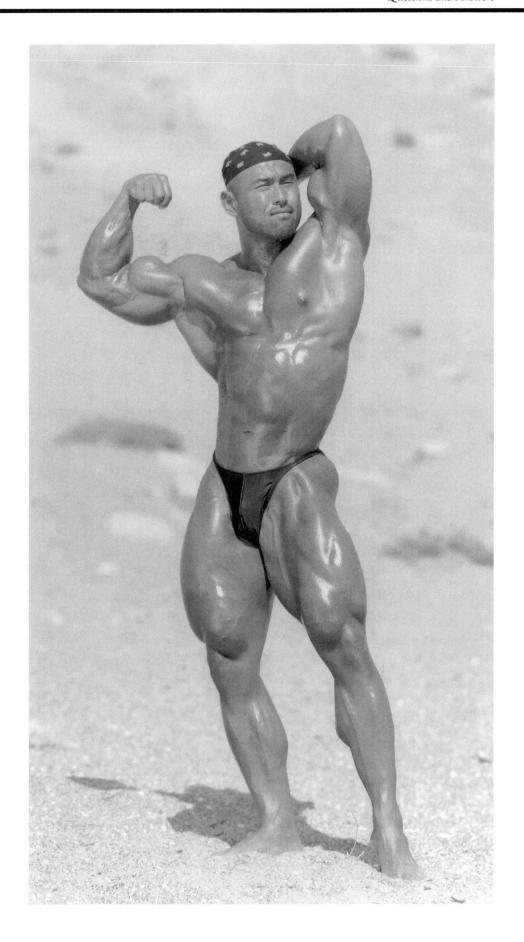

These workouts are extremely intense. The *only* way you can maintain this intensity is to do no other strength training whatsoever on your off days. It is very foreign to perform a workout that involves only 25 to 75 seconds of muscular work . . . but if you follow this program to the letter, you will see increases in strength that you never thought possible.

Remember, we have tested all of these parameters. We tried working people three times a week; it reduced results. We tried longer hold times; it reduced results. We tried more exercises; it reduced results. We tried extra sets; it reduced results. We tried mixing in full- and partial-range exercises; it reduced results. It's all about the intensity versus duration graph (see page 21); we have learned that *nothing* is more important than intensity! Sacrifice intensity in favor of anything and you will reduce your results.

Question: I want to do some experimentation with other exercises, but I'm not sure what part of the range of motion involves full contraction on some exercises—for example, leg extension, leg curl, and bent-over row.

Answer: It's always heartening to find out that people are willing to experiment with new applications to their training. Remember that the objective of any exercise should be to provide maximal overload to the target muscle or muscle group. By definition, maximal overload will be achieved in the range of motion that permits you to handle the heaviest weight possible for that exercise. This is easy to see in exercises like dips, used to overload triceps. From a fully locked-out position, the point of maximal triceps overload will be out of lockout and down only an inch or two rather than at the point where your body is fully lowered and your hands are near your armpits. The same is true on a close-grip bench press, where the strongest range is the last few inches of reach.

The issue is a little more confused on an exercise like a lat pulldown. While it can be argued that maximal contraction in a lat pulldown occurs when the bar is pulled all the way to your chest, the problem is that in this position your elbows are also bent and your biceps are performing a significant amount of work to hold that position statically. As your biceps weaken, your elbows are forced to straighten and allow the bar to rise toward the end of your reach. However, during the first one to three inches of motion in the lat pulldown, the biceps perform virtually none of the work of lowering the bar. Holding the weight statically in this part of the range will produce a fatigue in the lats that has to be felt to be believed. We have always seen the best progress in lat development when using this technique. When experimenting with any new exercise, just remember—maximal overload will occur when you are in a position that allows the maximum weight to be used in any exercise.

Question: Can Static Contraction Training be performed more often than conventional training?

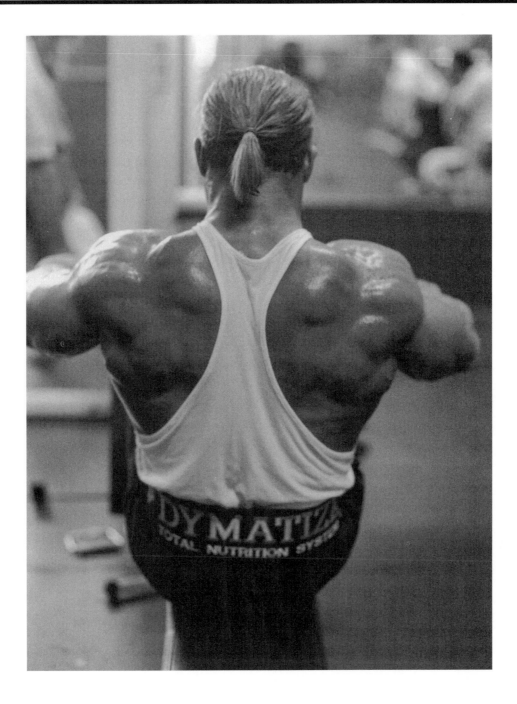

Answer: It seems likely (we have not conducted a formal study) that static contraction workouts could be performed more frequently than other workouts because the volume of work in a static contraction workout is much less. However, in many ways this would mitigate the value of the Static Contraction Training breakthrough. There are two sides to the issue of training frequency. One question for researchers is what is the greatest frequency of training that a body can withstand? Twice a week? Three times a week? Three and a half times a week? The other side of the issue is how infrequently can one perform a workout and either increase or maintain muscle mass? Static Contraction Training belongs to the realm of the latter question. The research we have done and will continue to do in the area of strength training will focus on how brief a workout can be in order to produce results, and how far apart those same workouts can be spaced in order to meet the objectives of growth and maintenance of muscle mass.

On the other hand, conventional training—particularly our own method of Power Factor Training—concerns itself with a higher volume of training (such as four sets of 20 reps) and is better suited to discovering the maximum tolerance of exercise both in volume and frequency. Please note that when we say volume we are referring to a very specific volume of high-intensity muscular output and not high volume at lower intensities, which we already know to be grossly inefficient, sometimes to the point of zero effectiveness.

Think of Static Contraction Training concerning itself with the question what is the minimum dose of exercise that will stimulate muscle growth? Power Factor Training concerns itself with the question what is the maximum dose of exercise the body can generate and tolerate?

Question: What are your thoughts on "super slow" reps?

Answer: Utilizing super slow reps (a technique that has been variously described as taking 10 seconds to one minute or more per rep) will stimulate muscle growth. The drawbacks of the technique are:

- If there is a full range of motion involved, then a lighter weight must be used in order for it to be manageable in the weakest range.
- Whenever a weight is being lowered, you can never be sure how hard you are pressing against that weight. For example, when a bar weighs 200 pounds and you are lowering it (super slow or otherwise), all we know for certain is that you are not pressing up with 200 pounds of force. You may be pressing up with 199 pounds or with 170 pounds. In effect, lowering a weight gives you some amount of rest. So comparisons of intensity from workout to workout begin to get vague. That's not good.

Remember, the Static Contraction Research Study proved that significant gains in mass and strength can be achieved without ever operating in the weakest range of motion, and in fact without engaging in any movement whatsoever. We suspect that the greatest benefits achieved while performing super slow sets are garnered when the weight is held in the strongest range almost statically.

Question: What about performing one set to failure, followed by a negative, followed by a static hold? I've heard several people recommend this and claim they had good results.

Answer: We have no doubt that this technique will get results. The difficulty we have with strategies like this is that we always want to know which of the three components is contributing the most to the growth process. We know that a training program of one set to failure will stimulate muscle growth. We also know that a program of only negatives will stimulate muscle growth, as will a program of only static holds. While we're on the subject, we know that pre-exhaustion, super sets, sets of 100, and so on will also build muscle. So what would be your opinion of a program that counseled a set of 100, followed by a super set, followed by a pre-exhaust, followed by one set to

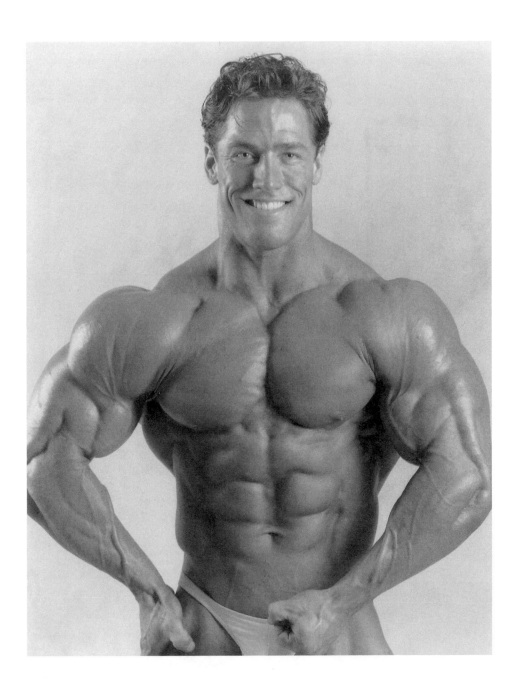

failure, then a negative, then a static hold? What would be your motivation for wanting to try a program like this? Are you interested in testing the limits of your tolerance to exercise? The fact is that any time you go into the gym, your body is capable of stimulating only *x* amount of growth, but no more. (Possibly less, but no more.) So wouldn't you be interested in the most efficient way of getting that *x* amount of growth? If a static hold will deliver your *x* amount of growth, why do more?

Question: When is a static rep finished?

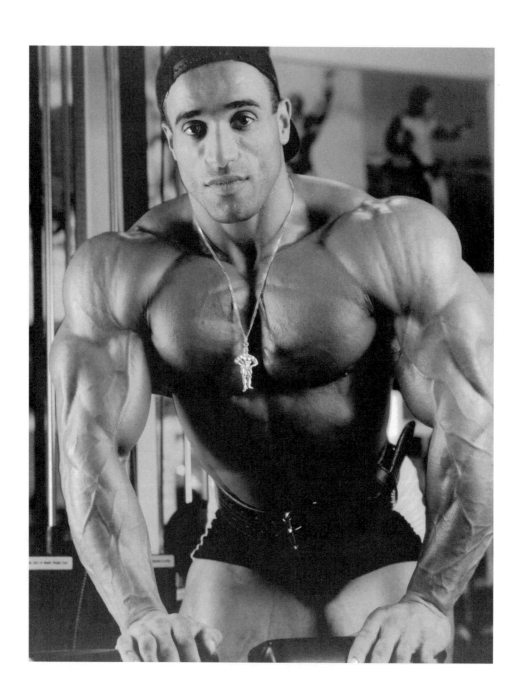

Answer: The objective of statically holding a weight is to hold the weight motionless in space. Once the weight begins to descend, the rep is over. This is an important distinction to make because, as mentioned earlier, when a weight is descending, all we know for certain is that you are pushing with insufficient force to hold the weight stationary. But we do not know exactly how insufficient. One pound? Ten pounds? Leaving the clock running during this period of unknown measurement would greatly sacrifice precision. The clock stops when the weight starts to drop.

Question: Doesn't the law of specificity of training mean that static contraction exercise cannot yield increases in full-range strength?

Answer: This is a very common belief that many people feel is supported by a valid theory. The specific adaptation to imposed demands (SAID) principle of physiology is valid and well established. Briefly, that principle states that the body will adapt itself in a manner that is appropriate to the demands or stress placed upon it. It should be noted, however, that this law states that there will be a specificity of adaptation but *not* an exclusivity of adaptation. If the body responded with an exclusive adaptation to imposed demands (EAID?), then a person who lifted weights through a full range of motion for many years would have no static strength whatsoever because he never imposed a static demand on his muscles. The converse would also be true; a person who trained for many years with only static contractions and was very muscular would be incapable of moving the lightest weight through any range of motion. It is obvious that the body does not operate this way. While there is conclusive evidence of a *specificity* of adaptation, it is by no means an *exclusivity*. Corroboration of this can be seen in our own SCRS, where subjects on average had a 60 percent increase in static strength over a 10-week period but "only" a 27.6 percent and 34.3 percent increase in their full-range dynamic strength of 1RM and 10RM. So the imposed demand of static contractions provided an increase in strength that was more specific to static strength than to dynamic strength.

The question for inquiring bodybuilders who have never tried a static contraction program should be whether they have seen a 27.6 to 34.3 percent increase in their dynamic strength during their last 10 weeks of conventional training. If they have not, they should consider switching to Static Contraction Training.

Question: Has there ever been a study proving that a full range of motion is necessary in order to stimulate muscle growth?

Answer: No. And there never will be. It may seem as though we are recklessly predicting the outcome of future scientific experiments by saying that there never will be a study that proves a full range of motion is necessary to stimulate muscle growth. In fact, however, we are correct with the highest order of certainty. First of all, our own experience with static contractions revealed that exercising with zero range of motion would stimulate substantial new muscle growth and strength increases. You cannot have one valid study that says zero range will stimulate muscle growth and a second valid study that says only 100 percent range of motion will stimulate growth.

Secondly, outside of the gym virtually none of the six billion people on the planet uses a full range of motion when going about their daily activities, and yet these people are all able to increase their muscle mass. For example, climbing stairs will increase the strength in your legs even though a six-inch step is nowhere near a full range of leg motion. It is perfectly rational to conclude that there never will be a study to conclude that a full range of motion is a requirement for muscle growth, just as there will never be a study proving that eating kiwi is a requirement for muscle growth.

Question: I've read in bodybuilding magazines that by training a muscle group from several different angles, you'll be bringing more mus-

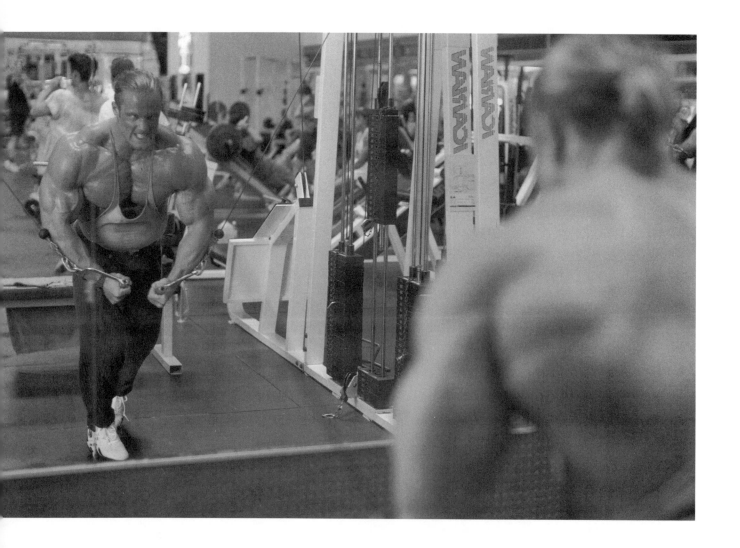

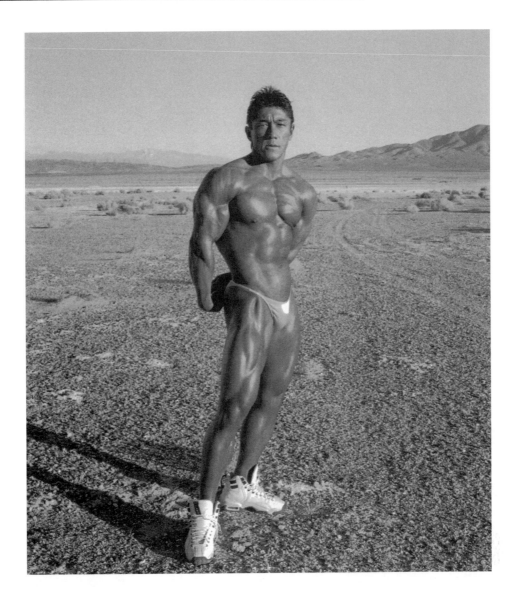

cle fibers into play that would not have been activated otherwise. For example, in order to hit all of the muscle fibers in my pecs, I should use flat bench presses to stress the outer portion of the pecs, incline presses to stress the upper portion of the pecs, and decline presses to hit the lower portion of the pecs. This seems to make perfect sense, so why don't you guys advocate angle training with your static contraction method?

Answer: There is no scientific basis for believing that more muscle fibers are "recruited" by training a muscle group from different angles. Moreover, if it were possible to limit the effective stress of focus to only one region of a muscle group, you would ultimately reduce the potential fiber involvement of the exercise and, hence, its productivity. The only factor that dictates muscle-fiber activation is how *heavy* the weight is—not the angle through which it's lifted. The heavier the weight, the more fibers are recruited to lift it, meaning that

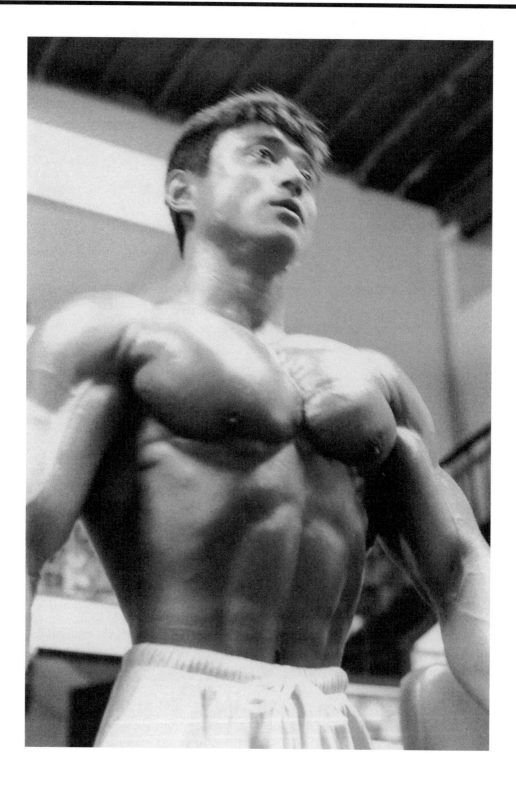

more fibers are stimulated to grow. Even if multiangle training could effectively isolate certain sections of a given muscle, doing so would limit the amount of fibers involved in a contraction and thereby reduce the amount receiving growth stimulation. This should not be any bodybuilder's objective. For example, if incline presses could stress only the upper pecs (which they don't), then you would be stimulating only one-third of your pectorals. You

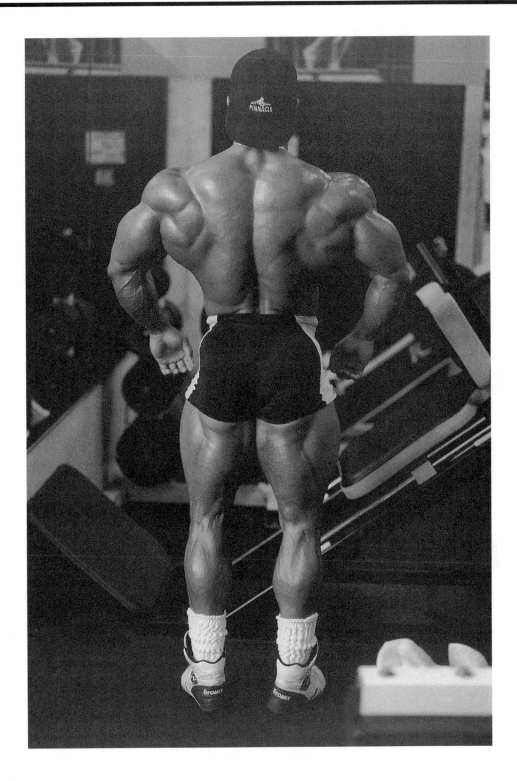

would need to perform additional pec work to stimulate the remaining two-thirds of your pecs. In other words, you would have to perform three exercises to stimulate one muscle complex. This would be a monumental waste of time—particularly because the upper and lower portions of the pec share a common tendon of insertion. This means that the fibers in both regions are activated whenever the muscle complex is called into play.

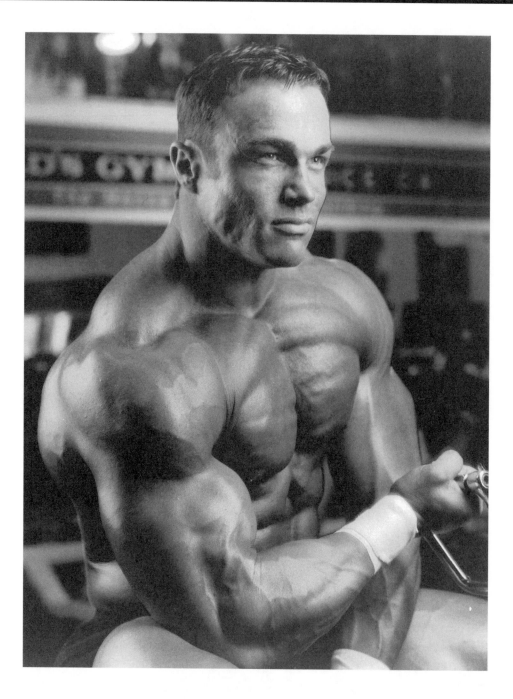

Question: Is it better to use machines or free weights in my Static Contraction Training?

Answer: It really makes no difference because muscles can't differentiate between a barbell, a Nautilus machine, or a bucket of rocks. It is only important that enough fibers are recruited to move the resistance you happen to be training with. In addition, exercises that allow you to contract against the heaviest weights possible will be the ones that will involve the most muscle fibers (such as the exercises suggested in the workouts in this book).

Question: I've read that since muscles adapt quickly to the stress of exercise, you've got to constantly change your exercises, sets, reps—even training systems—in order to keep your muscles "confused." Since they are confused, they cannot become complacent, and the constant change literally shocks your muscles into new spurts of growth. Is this true?

Answer: From a scientific standpoint, you cannot shock or confuse a muscle into doing anything but contract. Contraction is the singular function of muscle; therefore, performing a different exercise cannot be considered shock. For example, say you normally perform curls with a dumbbell. You won't "shock" your biceps muscle by switching to a barbell because the muscle will still be performing its primary function—contraction. Likewise you cannot "confuse" your muscle by changing the position from which you do an exercise. For example, the biceps muscle will contract regardless of whether you perform a dumbbell curve from a sitting or lying position.

Question: For years machine companies like Nautilus have advocated the performance of full-range exercise in order to create a fuller muscle. In fact, their offset cams were said to be "revolutionary." If I understand you correctly, you're saying that the Nautilus principles and, indeed, their machines are unnecessary.

Answer: We've never said that machines such as Nautilus are "unnecessary"; however, since a full range of motion does little for building maximum strength, the need for any training principles that advocate full-range exercise must be seriously questioned. Some machine companies, for example, maintain that if you perform full-range curls on one of their machines, the stress of the exercise will be more "directly focused" onto your "lower" biceps (then, of course, you'd have to buy one of their other biceps machines in order to train the remaining portions of your biceps). This is ridiculous; muscle fibers, regardless of where they are located in a given muscle, are recruited by one thing and one thing only—the amount of weight they are being made to contract against. All of the available muscle fibers in your biceps will be stimulated to grow bigger and stronger simply by employing a heavy enough resistance to recruit them all. Excessive stretching or an exaggerated range of motion plays no part at all in the muscle fiber recruitment process.

Question: I like to perform a heavy basic compound exercise for mass, another movement for shape, and a third for bringing out definition in my muscles. What's wrong with that?

Answer: You cannot train for shape or definition more successfully with isolation exercises than you can with compound exercises. In fact, there is no such thing as a "pure shaping" or a "pure definition" exercise. Heavy basic compound movements not only build muscle mass; they *also* bring out the inherent shape of your muscles *and* burn away body fat, thus leading to a more "defined" state. The burning of calories beyond what you consume in the form of calories is what will lead to definition, and heavy basic compound movements burn the most calories on a per set basis and will thus result in the greatest definition.

Question: While I like the idea of performing static contractions to build mass, I want to reduce my waistline. To this end, I've read that performing such abdominal exercises as twists with just an empty bar across my shoulders will reduce my waistline quite effectively. What are your thoughts on this?

Answer: Twists with an empty barbell across your shoulders will do absolutely nothing to reduce your waistline. The reason is that the movement does not offer appreciable resistance even when performed at a quick cadence. The waist or, more specifically, your obliques receive no training effect from the exercise. Nor, for that matter, does the movement use up enough calories to burn any fat. The loss of body fat is a systematic process; that is, you lose fat randomly from throughout the body—and even then only if you've burned significantly more calories through activity than you've taken in through food. When you go on a diet, fat is mobilized from all the body's multiple fat cells, not from isolated areas, such as the waist. Once fat has been broken down and mobilized, it is transported by the blood to all the individual active cells in the body and burned for energy. The only way to get rid of fat from around your obliques is to go on a calorie-reduced diet, and if you stay on it long enough, you'll eventually burn up all the fat in that area. In order to trim your waist and hasten the body's general fat-burning process, we recommend that you perform some form of aerobic activity, such as cycling, walking, jogging, or swimming. Your Static Contraction Training (which will increase your supply of lean muscle tissue) combined with aerobic activity will trim your waist and assist in keeping the fat from returning.

Question: For decades, many bodybuilding authors and even a few exercise physiologists have indicated that weight training "tears down the muscles" and that you should take a few days off in order to allow the muscles to build back bigger and stronger. Is this actually what happens?

Answer: While it may sound plausible, in reality, it just doesn't happen this way. Exercise performed for the express purpose of getting stronger, should never "tear down" or damage muscles. If it did, you wouldn't be able to leave

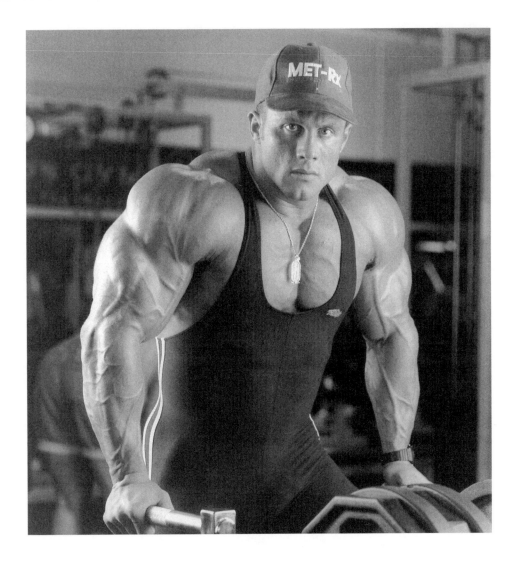

the gym after an intense weight workout. Proper bodybuilding training is geared to stimulate growth, not cause cellular trauma. In other words, the workout acts as a trigger mechanism that sets into motion a series of physiological steps that will, hopefully, culminate in the production of muscle growth—provided that certain preconditions, such as time for complete recovery and growth, are allowed to take place and adequate nutrition is consumed. While there will be some changes in muscle cell permeability as a result of an intense workout (often times a leakage of certain enzymes through the cell membrane can occur), there should never be dramatic alterations in the structural integrity of muscle fibers as a result of working out.

Question: I know many bodybuilders who say that "getting a good pump" is the only key to muscle growth stimulation. If this is so, then why all this talk of heavy weights?

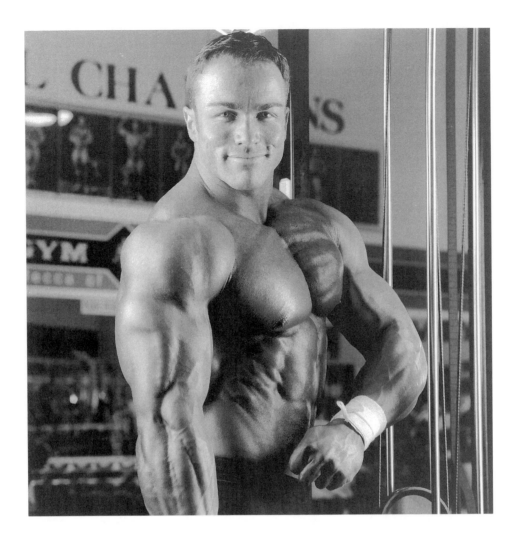

Answer: Simply because it isn't so. There exists no evidence whatsoever that a pump stimulates muscle growth. All bodybuilders achieve a pump to some degree every time they work out, yet, obviously, not all bodybuilders grow as a result of each workout. A pump is simply an edema, or a temporary swelling of tissue due to a fluid buildup—in this case blood—in the muscle being worked. Unless growth was stimulated as a result of a workout, however, the muscle will revert to its previous size once the pump has subsided. Strength training, which is what proper bodybuilding really is, doesn't always produce much in the way of a pump. Yet there can be no mistaking the fact that the body does undergo profound physiological changes after a hard peak overload workout. And therein lies the only true key to muscle growth as it was discovered a long, long time ago: muscular size and strength are directly related. In other words, a stronger muscle is a bigger muscle. For example, an injured limb will atrophy, or become smaller, while it is in a cast because it cannot be used. What's the doctor's prescription for rehabilitating that limb? To get those muscles to grow bigger again? Strength training! And the stronger the limb becomes, the bigger it becomes. In conclusion, if you want to grow bigger and bigger muscles, you should always train with an eye toward a strength improvement. A pump, while a nice feeling admittedly, is not an accurate indicator of muscle growth stimulation.

Question: I see plenty of bodybuilders training six days a week—and they're huge. So, why shouldn't I train every day if I want to?

Answer: Almost every professional bodybuilder is on some form of growth drug, which allows them to train so frequently without overtraining. However, growth drugs have dire side effects, which is why we adamantly oppose their use. We are concerned solely with the training requirements of human beings with *normal* human endocrinology, and what we've discovered is that *nobody* whose goal is making size and strength gains needs to train that frequently. Heavy overload exercise—the only kind that results in immediate muscular adaptation—is a form of stress to the muscles and the overall physical system. When performed properly such training will stimulate a compensatory buildup in the form of additional muscle size and strength that aids the body in coping more successfully with similar stressors in the future. However, bodybuilders who insist on training six to seven days a week will witness a decompensatory effect as the drain on the regulatory subsystems of the body will actually prevent the buildup of muscle tissue. In fact, all the energy reserves will have to be called upon simply to attempt to overcome the energy debt caused by such overtraining. These facts strongly indicate that the less time spent in the gym, the better your results will be. You'll find that your results will be spectacular if you limit your total training time to one, two, or—at the most—three workouts per week of roughly 45 to 60 minutes per session. Sufficient recovery time between workouts is vital.

Although recovery time will vary from individual to individual, most people starting out require a minimum of 48 hours between workouts in order to recover and grow stronger. However, as the trainee grows stronger, his body will be able to handle even *less* training before becoming overtrained and catabolic. The time needed between workouts in order for complete recovery and growth manifestation varies widely between individuals. After identical workouts, one person may be able to return to the gym in 48 hours and see an improvement in his strength, while another individual may need as many as eight weeks before his body recovers sufficiently and shows an increase in strength.

You should thus space your workouts by identifying both the first and last days that you can return to the gym and expect to see an improvement in strength. When there is no evidence of increased strength, your body is signaling that it needs time to recover. Regardless of what your personal range of recovery happens to be, one thing is certain—everyone's personal recovery ability takes much longer to replenish itself than was once thought. Training more than three days a week—and maybe even more than once a week—is going to be a mistake for most bodybuilders looking to increase their muscle mass.

[handwritten margin note: (?) Don't agree / some possess special genetic trait]

Question: I've been thinking of adding amino-acid supplements to my diet in an effort to further enhance recovery ability. What will they do for me?

Answer: The history of amino-acid supplements can be traced back to a time when protein supplements had become commercially less popular with the bodybuilding community due to scientific information disseminated by biochemists, physiologists, and nutritionally informed bodybuilders. They insisted that a well-balanced diet provided more than enough protein for the aspiring bodybuilder and that supplements were, by and large, a waste of money and the body's energy in digesting them. At this point, the protein manufacturers, in an attempt to recapture the tremendously lucrative protein market, reissued the old protein supplements—only this time with a new name—"amino acids." It's an example of old wine in new skins, as amino acids are simply the nitrogen-based constituents of protein and, consequently, yield the same "recovery enhancing" effect as their soy, milk, egg, and beef predecessors. Of course, not only did the labels have to change in order to market this "new" product, but also the marketing strategies employed to promote them had to as well. As a result, amino-acid supplements were touted by ad campaigns as safe, effective, and even superior replacements to anabolic steroids—which is tantamount to telling a man who is testosterone-deficient that all he needs is a good protein shake in order to set things right. It was at once obvious that such claims were ludicrous; after all, protein is a nutritional element, whereas a steroid is a hormone. There exists no similarity between the two. While one is a dietary consideration, the other is a drug—and there's a big difference between the two.

Amino acids *are* absolutely necessary for proper bodily and muscular function (including muscle growth); however, it makes no difference to your body whether they are in the form of a capsule, a pill, or a T-bone steak. Your body simply breaks down the macromolecule of protein into its constituent amino acids and redistributes the individual amino acids to where they're needed most. Each amino acid retains its distinctive chemical structure in order to be utilized to make up the varied sequences and structures of human proteins. Moreover, the body needs specific amounts of protein, and any additional amounts, such as those obtained through supplements, serve *no* biological value. As long as the cells have all the amino acids they need, regardless of how they were consumed, additional amino acids will not be put to work. Thus, making more amino acids available through supplements will not make cells multiply or renew at a faster rate.

The genes that shape our bodies—and particularly our muscular development—provide each cell with precise instructions for making proteins from amino acids. A small change in amino-acid sequence or structure can make a protein unusable—or even lethal. The method by which the trillions of cells in the human body encode and use this information has been known since the 1962 Nobel prize-winning discovery made by the scientists James Watson, Maurice Wilkins, and Francis Crick. This discovery revealed how a tiny amount of DNA in every cell carried the instructions for making the more than

100,000 proteins of the body. These cells use the instructions to determine what proteins have to be made and then signal that information to the chromosomes in the nucleus.

DNA itself is a chain of nucleotides, each of which is made of sugar, a phosphate, and a base. It's the sequencing of the nucleotides in DNA that actually instructs the cells to make the various proteins that the body needs. The DNA nucleotides are made partly from a sugar called *deoxyribose*, from which DNA takes its name. The chains which these nucleotides eventually make up are known as *ribonucleic acids* or RNA. Because RNA relentlessly seeks out amino acids only and because we know that all molecules of any one amino acid are completely interchangeable, we can conclude that the food source of the amino acids does not matter for protein synthesis. For example, if the DNA "blueprint" calls for the amino acid lysine, the transfer RNA will seek lysine and nothing else, without concern for whether that lysine molecule comes

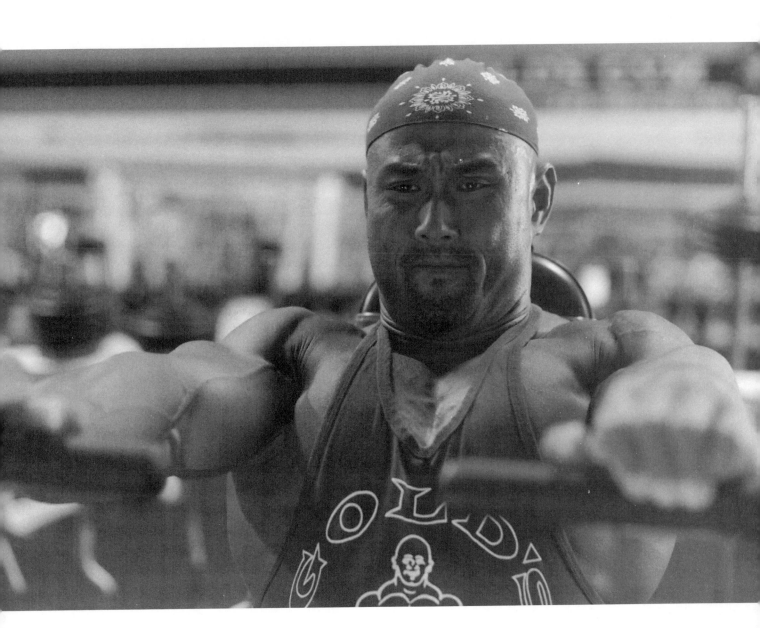

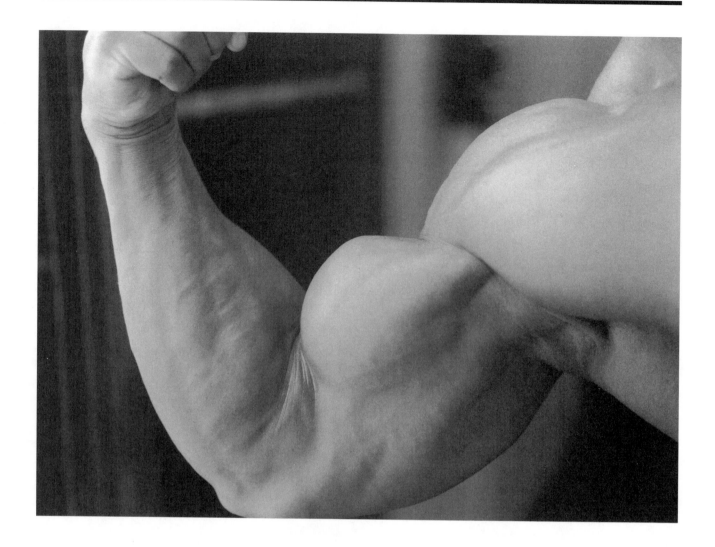

from a hot dog, a can of tuna, sunflower seeds, soy sprouts, or an amino-acid supplement. There is evidence, however, that we really do much better when the amino acids come from food rather than from supplements. It has been found that pure amino acids taken by mouth are not that well-absorbed. When liquid foods (which are used for patients with digestive problems) are formulated with a mix of some pure amino acids and short chains of amino acids, there seems to be better absorption.

Amino acids are not a requisite for building big muscles. To build big muscles you must first stimulate muscle growth at the cellular level via peak overload training and then allow sufficient time to elapse between workouts in order to allow your muscular reserves time to recover and grow. Then and only then does nutrition become a factor in the growth process. Adequate intake of *all* essential nutrients—not just protein or amino acids—must be provided in order for you to maintain your existing level of muscle mass, and if you stimulated growth by training with sufficient overload, a little bit extra (approximately 16 calories with a protein breakdown of .9 grams per kilogram of body weight) must be consumed in order to allow that growth to manifest.

A well-balanced diet consists of two or more portions of what was formerly known as the *Four Basic Food Groups*:

- Cereals and grains
- Fruits and vegetables
- Meats
- Dairy products

Food from these four groups, consumed daily, will provide you with sufficient nutrition to both maintain your health and—if you've stimulated it—allow for the growth of additional muscle mass. However, there is no way that amino-acid supplements themselves can either stimulate or accelerate the muscle growth process.

Question: Don't advanced bodybuilders rely on the "instinctive training" principle to make advanced gains?

Answer: Advanced bodybuilders rely on a good many things (many of them illegal) to make "advanced" gains. However, attempting to monitor one's results by such a subjective index as how one felt inclined to train at a given time yields nothing in the end. Only in bodybuilding could one postulate such a ludicrous hypothesis as "instinctive training" and get away with it. Could you imagine, for example, an Olympic sprinter trying to monitor his progress by feel or instinct instead of using a stopwatch? What if this sprinter had no tangible, objective measure of the effects of his training techniques or of his improvement from one month to the next? It's unthinkable! And yet this is exactly the kind of irrational, low-tech methodology that bodybuilders have always used. *Feeling* something to be true is no guarantee that it is true.

Question: I'm told that if my muscles get bigger, I'll become slower. Is this true?

Answer: The speed of a body movement is dependent on two factors:

- The strength of the muscles that are actually involved when performing a specific skill
- Your capacity to recruit muscle fibers while performing the movement (neurological efficiency)

It's fallacious to assume that a muscle will "slow down" if its strength and size increase. The correlation between the speed of a muscle movement and the strength level of the muscle are positively related. Therefore, to increase the speed of a muscle movement, increase the strength levels of the muscles needed to perform that particular movement.

Question: If I build a lot of muscle mass, won't it all turn to fat when I get older?

Answer: This is perhaps the most common misconception about proper bodybuilding. Muscle can no more be turned into fat than an apple can be turned into an orange; muscle and fat are two entirely different cells—one cannot "become" the other. If you were to chemically analyze fat and muscle, you would discover that muscle and fat both contain varying amounts of protein, water, lipids, and inorganic materials. However, when muscle is exercised, it contracts and produces movement, whereas fat will not contract and is usually stored in the body as a source of fuel. It is physiologically and chemically impossible to convert a muscle to fat and vice versa. A simple explanation of what *does* take place can be illustrated by observing an ex-athlete's pattern of exercise and caloric intake. When the athlete stops training his muscles, the muscles will begin to atrophy from disuse. At the same time, the athlete continues consuming the same level of calories. If the athlete is consuming more calories than are needed to maintain his body weight/energy demands, the excess will then be stored in the body as additional fat. Thus, if an athlete becomes obese after terminating a strength-training program, it is due to caloric imbalance—taking in more calories than are being burned off. Some individuals believe that their body weight should maintain a constant level upon the termination of a strength-training program. Unfortunately, these individuals fail to understand that if they lose 10 pounds of muscle mass through muscle atrophy and their body weight remains the same, then the weight loss that is attributed to muscle atrophy has been replaced by deposits of additional fat. In conclusion, upon stopping training, one should also alter his calorie intake.

Question: Won't "motionless exercise," such as Static Contraction Training, place inordinate stress on my joints and connective tissues?

Answer: Properly performed, Static Contraction Training, using what for you are "heavy" weights, will actually *strengthen* the muscles surrounding each joint, making the joint more stable and less susceptible to injury. In fact, proper overload on the ligaments and tendons in the joint region actually serves to thicken and therefore strengthen them (much the same as a callus forming on the hands). Far from being a potential danger, Static Contraction Training is probably the safest manner in which an individual can train. A greater potential for injury lies, not in performing heavy static holds (which we advocate being performed in the body's most advantageous leverage and muscular range), but rather in full-range movements that can weaken the joints and connective tissues by exceeding (often considerably) their structural integrity. Extreme stretching of joints can cause very real damage to ligaments and tendons.

Question: When should I return to full-range training?

Answer: This question is often asked by people on Power Factor and Static Contraction Training. The fallacy inherent in this question is the presupposition that there is some advantage to returning to full-range training and some disadvantage to training in an unconventional manner.

Let's take a look at what we've learned in the last five years or so. In 1992 we undertook the task of finding a more efficient way to exercise for increased muscle mass and strength gains. Using a Power Factor and Power Index measurement in order to quantify the intensity of various techniques, we discovered that strong-range partial repetitions generated not only the highest overload but also garnered tremendous results in both size and strength gains. Thus, Power Factor Training was born and introduced in 1993 in the book of the same name. In that first edition we recommended that trainees perform reps exclusively in the strongest range, which we recommended as four to six inches of motion for most movements. As PFT gained worldwide popularity, we began to get feedback from the 20,000 people in 58 countries who were training on and experimenting with this new system. It came as no surprise to us that these trainees experienced the same remarkable results as we had during its development. (It should be noted that the very few letters and calls we did receive from people who made either no progress or initial progress followed by no progress did, without exception, ignore their PF and PI calculations. In effect, these were the people who replace conventional overtraining with strong-range partial overtraining. They wrongly considered PFT to be about partials and nothing more.) What did surprise us was the number of people who informed us that they had reduced their range of motion to two and even one inch of up-and-down motion and were reporting the best results they'd ever experienced. This caused us to wonder how important range of motion could be, if at all.

John Little had done preliminary experimentation with static contractions approximately 10 years earlier, but had never fully analyzed his data or published his findings. Together we constructed a research study that would measure the effects of zero range of motion training on size and strength gains throughout a full spectrum of exercises. The results of that study proved that very substantial gains could be made, even with experienced weightlifters who were nearing middle age. The conclusive evidence was that the range of motion has virtually no importance in attaining size and strength gains. The fact is that greater gains can be made by holding a very heavy weight stationary in the strongest range than can be made by moving a lighter weight through a full range of motion. Since a greater range of motion has no benefit, what would be the argument for using a lighter weight through a full range of motion?

We cannot overemphasize the importance of this last point, as it is destined to change strength training for all time. Those of you reading this are privy to a piece of information that has gone completely unrecognized in the world of exercise physiology. It is our earnest belief that at some point in the future, be it 2 years, 20 years, or 50 years from now, strength training will be almost unrecognizable from today's routines. Conventional thinking is wrong on the range of motion required, wrong on the duration of training required, and wrong on the frequency of training required. In the future a person wishing to maintain lean mass will probably lift weights statically with a total workout time of one minute or less performed with about the same frequency as getting a haircut.

When should you return to conventional training? On the same day you decide to leave your car in the garage and ride a horse to work.

Question: I want to gain muscle and lose fat. Can I mix cardiovascular workouts with strength workouts and not overtrain?

Answer: This is another of the most common questions we receive. The lack of good information on this subject still continues to amaze us. Aerobic training to lose fat is vastly different than efficient anaerobic training to gain strength. There is really no reason to abandon one in favor of the other. Aerobic training, by definition, is low intensity and of an extended duration. This means that if you are jogging on a treadmill, for example, that you should be able to carry on a normal conversation with the person beside you. You should not be gasping for breath or otherwise exerting yourself at a rate you cannot sustain for 20, 30, or 40 minutes. This type of low-intensity exercise has wonderfully beneficial effects on the cardiovascular system, but does virtually nothing to tax the skeletal muscles. While it can always be argued that the body has a finite recovery capacity and that any exercise other than weightlifting will decrease your rate of progress, we have yet to see a single person arrest his strength-training progress by performing aerobics three or four days per week. It should be noted that the progressive intensity that is critical to anaerobic strength training is not a required element of aerobic training. The inability to make this distinction causes some bodybuilders to engage in "progressive aerobics" that eventually sees them donning 40-pound backpacks and running hills in order to outdo their last effort. That is not proper aerobic training. In aerobics it is entirely appropriate to adopt a program of, say, four 30-minute walks per week and then leave that program unchanged for 20 years. It's only when you turn your aerobic training into a high-intensity effort that it can begin to make any appreciable decrease in your rate of progress in strength training.

Question: My strength has gone up from training but my size has stayed the same. Should I be training differently?

Answer: The belief that there are separate ways to train for size and for strength is without any foundation in reality. There are many reasons why size gains do not manifest as quickly as strength gains. These reasons are due to the laws of both physiology and geometry. Think of it this way—if there were a method of training that delivered size gains without strength gains, it would be possible to develop enormous muscle size but still lack the ability to lift even the lightest weight. Similarly, if there were a way to train that would develop tremendous strength but no increases in size, then it would be possible to squat 800 pounds and bench 500 pounds with pencil-thin legs and arms. Obviously, this is not the way the human body functions. Muscle size and muscle strength share an exact correlation, and if you are getting appreciably stronger, then your muscles are getting bigger. Period.

The single greatest tool in helping you realize that you are making both strength and size gains at the same time is a set of skinfold calipers or another body-fat measuring device. Using a combination of a bathroom scale and calipers, you will discover that as you get stronger your lean mass is increasing. Without the calipers you might discover that although you got stronger, your weight decreased by five pounds and your arms don't look or measure any bigger. The truth, however, may be that you've gained 10 pounds of muscle, lost 15 pounds of fat (much from your arms), and are actually making terrific progress. Take the time to apply some reason and science to your training and you will be rewarded with the satisfaction of seeing your progress and staying motivated.

Question: How can I find out what you guys are working on right now?

Answer: We'll try to keep you updated on our Web page (www.precisiontraining.com).

Train Smart,
Pete Sisco
John Little

Index